# *Dementia with Dignity*

# Dementia with Dignity

## A GUIDE FOR CARERS
### SECOND EDITION

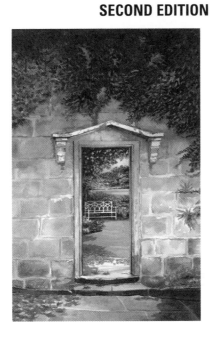

# Barbara Sherman

McGRAW-HILL BOOK COMPANY Sydney

New York  San Francisco  Auckland  Bogotá
Caracas  Lisbon  London  Madrid  Mexico City
Milan  Montreal  New Delhi  San Juan
Singapore  Tokyo  Toronto

# McGraw·Hill Australia

*A Division of The McGraw·Hill Companies*

Text © 1999 Barbara Sherman
Illustrations and design © 1999 McGraw-Hill Book Company Australia Pty Limited
Additional owners of copyright material are credited on the Acknowledgments page.

**National Library of Australia Cataloguing-in-Publication data:**

Sherman, Barbara.
Dementia with dignity : a handbook for carers.

2nd. ed.
Includes index.
ISBN 0 074 70752 3.

1. Dementia—Patients—Hospital care. 2. Dementia—Nursing. 3. Geriatric nursing. 4. Dementia—Patients—Long-term care. I. Title.

610.7365

Published in Australia by
**McGraw-Hill Book Company Australia Pty Limited**
**4 Barcoo Street, Roseville NSW 2069, Australia**
Acquisitions Editor: Kristen Baragwanath
Production Editors: Sybil Kesteven, Sarah Baker
Designer: Jenny Pace Design
Cover illustrator: Keith Scanlon
Illustrator: Alison Wallace, Lonely Badger Graphics
Technical illustrator: Alan Laver, Shelly Communication
Typeset in Berkeley by Jenny Pace Design
Printed on 80 gsm woodfree by Best Tri Colour Printing & Packaging Pty Limited, Hong Kong

# Bill

For a long time before Bill went to the nursing home, he had lived in an increasingly confused and frightening world. For much of the time his memory failed him completely. When his family and friends asked 'Do you remember?', he felt challenged and angry and would retort, 'Of course I do.' But he did not.

There were occasions, though, when he had clear flashes of memory and moments of inexplicable logic, or he would make an observation so penetrating that it was hard to believe his mind was failing.

Sport, politics, television, radio and other things that had previously interested him ceased to make much sense. Yet he gained endless pleasure from the songs he knew and loved and he effortlessly recalled most of the words.

Bill strenuously resisted help with dressing, but more often than not he could not remember which part of his body his socks or shirt fitted. He no longer knew about buttons, zippers and other fastenings. Knobs, handles and switches had no meaning. Even though he could name familiar objects, most times he did not know what to do with them. One day, he tried to eat his soup with a shoehorn, but then, sensing something was wrong, he broke down and cried.

Recurring hallucinations and delusions terrified him; there were nights when he believed the man who shared his room was collecting bodies. At other times he thought it was his turn to scrub the floor or that the staff used an electronic device to control his limbs.

Sometimes he seemed comforted by his perceptions. The movement nearby of what he saw as tanks and trucks at a US army camp (in reality, a freeway under construction) provided him with an endless talking point about his wartime experiences. And the water he 'heard' gurgling and bubbling from an imaginary hole in the floor under his bed satisfactorily explained away embarrassing incontinence.

There were other stories, too, which served to fill in the gaps in his memory and so helped him make sense of his 'nightmares'. So real did they seem and so convincingly vivid in detail were they that they caused conflict among the people around him. For example, his complaints about the nurse who stole his money and the patient who ate his chocolate. We would find the money, and sometimes the chocolate, where he had secreted them—in socks, ointment jars, or stuffed into slippers.

For a long time his family silently disapproved of the sympathetic doctor who, he insisted, wanted to look after him in her own home. On another occasion they looked for another nursing home because Bill had said, 'They can't keep me here any longer.'

Although they visited him every day, he would tell others 'My family hasn't been to see me for weeks … they've put me away and taken all my money.' At other times he would tell them, 'I'm packing now, they're taking me home today.'

A futile search by a lifelong friend followed Bill's demand to see his pet dog, which he said lived in a kennel in the nursing home garden.

A courteous man who had always been particular about his appearance, he was painfully aware of his degradation and inconsolable about his loss of dignity. Yet his whimsical sense of humour stayed with him until the end, as did his smile, so characteristic of the dementing—rare and beautiful.

Bill was my husband.

# Foreword

It is almost a decade since Barbara Sherman wrote the first edition of *Dementia with Dignity: A Handbook for Carers.* The book has been a great success as evidenced by a revised first edition, a videotape based on the book and now this second edition.

Since then the ageing of the population of the world has continued apace. In parallel with this demographic shift, Alzheimer's Disease International has published estimates that the number of people in the world with dementia will increase from 10.5 million in 1980, of whom 53 per cent were in the developing world, to 13.5 million in 2000, of whom 61 per cent will be in the developing world. By 2025 there will be 32 million people with dementia in the world, of whom 71 per cent will be in developing countries. In other words, by 2025 there will be twice as many people with dementia in the developed world as there were in 1980 and four times as many in the developing world."

In Australia almost 13.8 per cent of the population is now aged 65 years or more and 2.2 per cent is aged 85 years or greater. These percentages are set to pass 20 per cent and 8 per cent respectively by 2031, by which time the present population of 18.6 million will have surpassed 24 million. Community services for the elderly have grown and there has been modest growth in the number of beds in low care residential facilities (hostels), but not in high care residential facilities (nursing home), which have remained static at approximately 75 000. The previous ratio of 60 nursing home beds for every 1000 persons aged 70 years or more has been reduced to 40. The Commonwealth has capped growth in nursing homes and transferred the budget to the community and hostel sectors.

A consequence of these policies has been the change in the nature of residents in nursing homes. They are sicker, their dementia is more severe and the prevalence of behavioural disturbances is greater. Rates may be as high as 50 per cent for psychosis, 20 per cent for physically aggressive behaviour and 30 per cent for clinical depression.

There are many reasons for this staggering prevalence of behavioural and psychiatric symptoms of dementia, which can be abbreviated as BPSD. First, persons with dementia complicated by BPSD are significantly more likely to be admitted to a nursing home, as their families are less able to care for them at home. Second, as dementia advances almost all types of BPSD become more common and it is likely that the pathological changes in the brain are driving many of the disturbing behaviours. Third, changes in the environment, such as a lower standard of living, lack of privacy, loss of contact with familiar loved ones, interactions with other residents, may exert negative influences. Fourth, poorly managed BPSD may exacerbate the frustrations of professional as well as family carers which in turn may reduce their ability to cope and result in a positive feedback loop.

Behavioural and psychiatric symptoms are distressing to the person with dementia, to other residents, to the family and to the professional staff caring for the person in the residential facility. For example, BPSD account for about 25 per cent of the variance in family carer distress across many countries, for many types of dementia and regardless of whether distress is measured, as depression score, burden level or general psychological morbidity.

The management of BPSD is a challenge. Drug treatments have limited efficacy and are too broad in their actions. For example, antipsychotics are used to control aggressive behaviour, but they are not specifically designed for this purpose. Also, as with many psychotropic medications, antipsychotics have anticholinergic side effects, which may exacerbate the confusion experienced by people with dementia. Some of the newer medications hold more promise. Behavioural management strategies are more appealing and have empirical support. However they must be devised and applied by suitably qualified and trained professionals and their implementation requires staff time.

Periodic public outcries reveal evidence of mistreatment, over-sedation and illegal or inappropriate physical restraint in nursing homes. In the US, this led to federal guidelines about the prescribing of psychotropic medications. In New South Wales, Australia, sensational media stories in the newspapers and on television prompted an inquiry by the Social Issues Committee of the Legislative Council of the NSW Parliament, and a Ministerial Inquiry into the Use of Psychotropics in Nursing Homes. Both reports, (the Ministerial Inquiry has still not released despite a draft being circulated for comment in May 1997), contain important recommendations that if implemented should improve the standard of care in residential care.

Another highly significant development since the first edition of *Dementia with Dignity* is the advent of drugs to treat Alzheimer's disease. The importance of these drugs exceeds the modest but real gains they exert on cognitive and functional abilities. The previous nihilism that pervaded professional attitudes to dementia is now being replaced by a positive approach. General practitioners are more interested in early and accurate diagnosis of the cause of cognitive impairment. Pharmaceutical companies and clinicians are spurred to engage in research. Most gratifyingly, people with dementia and their carers now have hope that something can be done.

It will be some years before these advances produce a cure, a means to prevent Alzheimer's disease or the other dementias, or dramatic changes in the management of dementia. Until then, those in closest contact with persons with dementia continue to have the greatest impact on their quality of life. Kindness, humanity and a positive attitude are key to quality care but alone are insufficient. Knowledge and skill equip carers to understand and manage behaviours that seem unfathomable. Barbara Sherman's book does this wisely and practically. In plain language, generously illustrated with real-life examples derived from her decades of work in the field, Barbara explains what seems mysterious: the origins of the behaviours, the person behind the diagnosis and useful, humane strategies on how to help the person.

Henry Brodaty
Professor of Psychiatry of Old Age
University of New South Wales

Director, Academic Department of Psychiatry of Old Age,
Prince of Wales Hospital, Randwick, NSW, 2031

June 1999

# About the author

After graduating in Social Work from Sydney University Barbara Sherman worked as a researcher at the University's Institute of Child Health. She was later employed in a private organisation caring for multi-handicapped children and their parents, then as a Social Worker in Epidemiology in the NSW Department of Health. Following that, she worked at Gladesville Psychiatric Hospital as a field teacher in Social Work for the University of NSW, then as the Senior Social Worker.

When Barbara retired from the hospital she worked in a large retirement complex where she played a significant role in establishing one of the first dementia-specific units in Australia.

She has been widely published on the social aspects of mental illness and dementia and has always sought to promote a better understanding of the person with dementia. The first edition of *Dementia with Dignity* was published by McGraw-Hill in 1991. In 1998 ACER Press published her ground-breaking book *Sex, Intimacy and Aged Care*.

Since leaving the retirement complex in 1989 Barbara has pursued an eventful career as educator, consultant, lecturer and speaker on aged care. She has always worked passionately for the rights of people with mental illness and people with dementia, and for their families, and has served on many planning and policy making committees, within both the government and voluntary sectors. One of these was a Commonwealth Government committee which designed education programs for carers of people with dementia.

Barbara served as a wireless operator (Sergeant) in the Women's Australian Air Force in World War II. She is now an active member of the University of the Third Age and she teaches creative writing in a voluntary capacity. She has two daughters, four grandchildren and two great-grandchildren. Her husband suffered from Alzheimer's disease and Parkinson's disease.

# Contents

v BILL

vii FOREWORD

x ABOUT THE AUTHOR

xiii ACKNOWLEDGMENTS

1 INTRODUCTION

5 **CHAPTER ONE**
EXPLODING THE MYTHS

10 **CHAPTER TWO**
ABOUT DEMENTIA

16 **CHAPTER THREE**
ABOUT THE PERSON WITH DEMENTIA
17 *Memory loss*
23 *Confusion*
29 *Misunderstanding and misusing words*
34 *Difficulty in coordinating thoughts and actions*
43 *Delusions, hallucinations and confabulation*
49 *Walking and wandering*

55 **CHAPTER FOUR**
PERSONALITY AND MOOD CHANGES AND EMOTIONAL REACTIONS
55 *Changes in personality*
57 *Listlessness and depression*
62 *Emotional reactions*

68 **CHAPTER FIVE**
EACH PERSON IS UNIQUE
68 *Getting to know the person*
71 *Self-identity*
73 *Life-roles and habits*
78 *Humour, confabulation and social front*
81 *Ways to confirm identity*

**88 CHAPTER SIX**
**THE PROBLEM-SOLVING APPROACH TO HANDLING BEHAVIOUR**
94 *The problem-solving approach*

**101 CHAPTER SEVEN**
**FREQUENTLY OCCURRING PROBLEM BEHAVIOURS**
101 *Anger and aggression*
108 *Attention seeking—looking for love and care*
111 *Repetitiveness*
114 *Non-cooperation and negative reactions*
117 *Losing, hiding, accusing, rummaging, pilfering and giving away*
121 *Evening agitation and sleeplessness*
127 *Eating*
133 *Sexuality and sexual behaviour*
139 *Loss and grief*

**144 CHAPTER EIGHT**
**WORKER SKILLS**
144 *Communicating*
157 *The working relationship*
162 *Stepping into the person's world*
167 *Modelling*
169 *Reinforcement*
174 *Handling change*

**179 CHAPTER NINE**
**CARING**
179 *At home*
195 *Moving to a nursing home or hostel*
203 *Settling in*
212 *The residential facility*
218 *Life in the residential facility*
229 *Keeping occupied*
242 *Families*
247 *Staff—caring for yourself*

254 *Appendix A Personal profile*
256 *Appendix B Problem-solving approach*
258 *Appendix C The seven rules of caring for the home carer*
261 *Appendix D Carer support organisations*
263 *List of terms*
266 *Bibliography*
270 *Index*

# Acknowledgments

Many people contributed to the birth of this book in 1991. I am still indebted to the people who contributed to the original book: social work students from the University of New South Wales; participants in my interdisciplinary training sessions; staff in the Montefiore special care unit; the staff of Minna Murra Lodge, Toowoomba, Queensland; Dr Jillian Kril; Dr Tom Lonie; David Young, physiotherapist; Pam Jones and other colleagues; my publisher, McGraw-Hill, and in particular, John Rowe; Jenny Armstrong, then Senior Social Worker at the Royal Prince Alfred Hospital, for the time spent in reading the final draft. My editor at McGraw-Hill for this edition, Sybil Kesteven, has been a source of encouragement, patience and excellent suggestions which I have very much appreciated.

Jennie Hunt, then Support Group Coordinator, Alzheimer's Association NSW, suggested the title and provided the anecdote on Mr Peck in Chapter 7. Without Jennie's interest the book might not have been started.

Betty Wilkinson, my friend and social work colleague of many years, persistently encouraged me, week by week, patiently reading each section. Her long experience with and knowledge of the problems of brain-failed people and their relatives have been invaluable.

The idea 'look for the person behind the illness' I adapted from the concept of 'look behind the label', which was created by a group from the NSW Association for Mental Health for the project 'Taking the mystery out of mental illness', during the Year of the Disabled (1981).

In the intervening years I have met and listened to so many home carers, residential care workers and other professionals working with people with dementia all over Australia. I have visited countless dementia units and nursing homes. All of these have in some way contributed to this edition but to tell it all would take several volumes. Thank you.

To all those people with dementia and their families especially, whom I had the privilege of knowing and who taught me so much—thank you.

# Introduction

This is not a book about illness. It is about people.

The nicest thing about having written the first edition of *Dementia with Dignity* is that wherever I go in the world someone will come up to me and tell me how much it has helped them. While the original book was written with professional carers in mind, judging by the remarkable response from home carers, it has been of great benefit to them as well. They tell me first that it has helped to understand the strange ways their relative acts and their sometimes difficult behaviour, and has given them a choice of coping techniques that have been successful. Second, they say that it has given them insight into nursing homes and dementia hostels and an understanding of what they should expect from those residential facilities. I have emphasised home care more in this edition.

In this second edition I have maintained the format of the original book. The approach too is essentially the same—the personal approach—a philosophy that emphasises the humanistic belief that every person is a valued adult in his or her own right, despite the handicaps imposed by dementia. Also implied in this philosophy is the expectation that each person affected by a dementia illness will be treated with understanding, respect and courtesy. Also in keeping with this philosophy I have avoided using the current politically correct terms such as 'managing', 'controlling' and 'challenging' when referring to the behaviour of people affected by dementia. I believe that handicap and caring are about humanness and as such, these strong terms do not have a place.

I first wrote this book in the knowledge that people, even in the advanced stages of a dementing illness, can gain considerable enjoyment from life. I believe everyone is entitled to the best possible quality of life, to live in comfortable surroundings with dignity and the assurance that he or she is a worthwhile and valued individual.

A person in the early stages of a dementia illness is able to live a relatively normal life at home. In the final stages, tender loving care and understanding is what is most needed. In between, the disease progresses to more *advanced* stages, where the home carer experiences difficulty in managing and is unable to carry on alone. At this stage families seek help from community services, and permanent accommodation in a special hostel or nursing home is often necessary.

In the advanced stages of dementing illnesses, memory loss and confusion are severe, coordination of thoughts and actions is deteriorating and behaviour may be hard to understand and difficult to manage. As well, the person often realises memory is fading and confusion is increasing. This in itself can cause anxiety and depression.

New surroundings, particularly in the move from a home to a hostel or nursing home, aggravate these feelings. And, not fully comprehending what is happening, the person becomes frightened and may react with tears, hysterics, aggression and agitated pacing, and may try to run away to find family and home. By understanding these reactions and developing confidence to cope with a range of behaviours as they arise, both the home carer and the professional will be able to help new residents settle in and ensure they continue to have the best possible lifestyle.

Discover the person behind the illness! In cases of illness and disability, there is a tendency to think only of the symptoms and overlook the person. There is also a tendency to view people with dementia as being all the same, as a 'they' or a 'them' who all behave in the same way and have exactly the same needs. This belief can influence a disregard of the wide range of differences among dementing people, so hastening the loss of a person's identity—the sense of being 'me'. Even in the advanced stages, part of the adult personality is intact; it is not unusual for some skills, memories and a strong sense of humour to be retained.

To stress the need to consider each person as an individual in his or her own right, I have elected to talk about 'the person' and 'the resident' rather than 'patients' and 'clients', and where possible to use 'he' and 'she' rather than 'them' and 'they'.

Because of memory loss, confusion and failing capacity, there is a tendency to stress what the person cannot do, the deficits. Rather, we should stress the abilities still remaining, the strengths. By encouraging the person to use his or her remaining strengths, we help the person retain abilities a little longer and enhance feelings of being useful and wanted.

Much that has been written about dementing illness refers to Alzheimer's disease, the most commonly diagnosed; however, there are a number of dementia illnesses, the characteristics of which differ according to the specific illness. In this book I have covered a range of characteristics and behaviours that are likely to be experienced.

Some of the text is taken from transcripts of training sessions, lectures and talks to carers, and for easy reference I have tried to produce each section as complete in itself. Some repetition is, therefore, unavoidable.

The anecdotes used in the book are about real people. Many are taken from my personal experience, others from the experiences of my colleagues and of carers. Names are, of course, fictitious and composite examples have been used to further protect identities.

I hope that, in sharing with you the experiences and techniques that have been effective for me and others, I can inspire you to create your own way of working with the dementing person. By achieving this, your work will bring its own satisfaction and the lives of those in your care will be more enjoyable.

In attempting to retain the original text of *Dementia with Dignity*, while incorporating more information for the family carer, I have addressed professional workers and at times, the family carer. This is particularly so in the sections 'Caring at home', 'Moving into a nursing home' and 'Settling in'. However, the whole book is equally applicable to, and of interest to both groups of carers.

Like most people you are probably confused by the various terms generally given to family carers and professional carers. These are the terms usually used:

**Home carer** carer; family carer; primary carer; caregiver; relative; spouse

**Professional carer** care worker; worker; respite worker; respite carer; in-home respite carer; professional; professional worker; staff; personal care assistant; nurse; nurse assistant

**Other disciplines** doctor; social worker; psychologist; physiotherapist; gerontological nurse; practitioner; occupational therapist; recreation worker; diversional therapist.

# CHAPTER ONE

# Exploding the myths

Over the years many myths and misconceptions have grown up around dementia. These myths have influenced the way we feel and act towards people who suffer from dementing illnesses. Here we examine some of these myths.

## Myth

*'They're all the same.'*

People with dementia are *not* all the same, nor are they all affected in the same way. Just because people have similar illnesses it does not mean they will necessarily display the same symptoms. The way that any one person is affected by dementia depends on the part of the brain that is damaged by the disease and the particular disease that he or she suffers from. You will find that even people with the same illness may display different symptoms. People with dementia are still individuals, with distinctive personalities and ways of behaving.

## Myth

*'They're going through their second childhood. The kindest way to treat them is as though they are children.'*

People with dementia are *not* children. It is true that people with dementing illnesses, particularly those suffering from Alzheimer's disease, gradually unlearn what they previously knew as the brain fails. And, as the disease worsens, they become unable to do some of the things they used to be able to do. Until the disease reaches a severe stage, however, most still have a sense of being an adult with adult needs and feelings. Distress when they realise they are not coping is not unusual. To patronise such a person by treating them as a child will often create feelings of frustration and anger, and add to that distress.

# Myth

*'There's no point in telling them anything, because it won't register. It doesn't matter what you say in front of them because they won't understand.'*

Such remarks, often made in front of the person with dementia, can be hurtful. The person may well *understand* but not be able to *tell* you so. Always speak to or with the person, not about him or her.

# Myth

*'Outings such as films, excursions or birthday parties are a waste of time. They don't remember them.'*

You do not have to *remember* to enjoy. People with dementia have a great capacity for pleasure. If someone forgets an event, it does not mean it was not enjoyed at the time.

# Myth

*'It's a waste of money to buy them good clothes. They don't know/care how they look.'*

Many dementing people take pride in their appearance and have a clear picture of how they like to look. Some become even more particular about their clothes and hygiene than they were before they contracted the disease.

It is true, however, that some do lose interest in themselves and, if left to their own devices, become untidy and scruffy. On occasions this may happen because they cannot tell people how they would like to look. But there is no reason for them not to be nicely dressed in their own clothes.

# Myth

*'You need to lock them up or restrain them, otherwise they wander away and get lost.'*

Not everyone wanders away and gets lost, or has a tendency to do so. Where the route is familiar, some people are capable of going out alone and finding the way back. People who are used to freedom and understand that they are being restricted become frustrated and may try to escape.

However people who are at risk of wandering away need to be accommodated in secure areas with ample space for walking.

# Myth

*'Don't bother to give them things. They don't know they've got them and will only lose them anyway.'*

It is important for the person with dementia to have as many familiar objects as possible around them to see and to feel. Possessions are part of a person. They are part of the body image and identity and give a feeling of security.

In nursing homes or hostels, it is better that the articles are not of great sentimental or monetary value, so that if they are temporarily mislaid, no great harm is done.

# Myth

*'Don't let them have buttons/scissors/spoons/tools. They'll injure themselves or may attack another person.'*

Only a few dementing people will use articles harmfully. Even when an object is inappropriately 'tasted', it is seldom swallowed. As long as someone can handle familiar tools or implements without risk, they should be encouraged to do so.

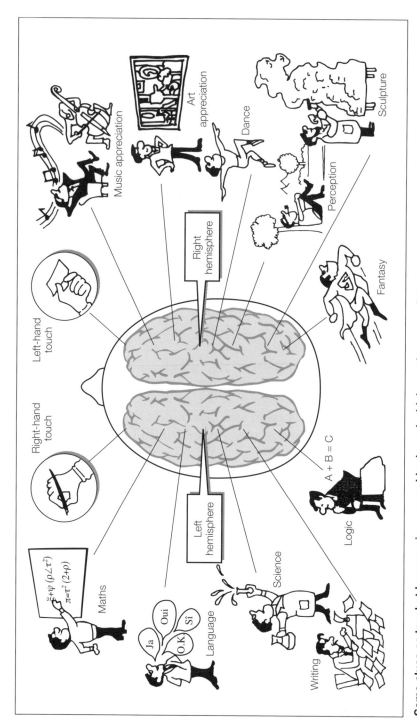

**Some clues as to what happens in a normal brain and which part is responsible for what.**
ADAPTED FROM ADARDS NSW NEWSLETTER, 9 JULY/SEPTEMBER 1988

# Myth

*'Very brainy people are more at risk of becoming demented than those who are less bright.'*

Intelligent people are no more at risk of being affected by dementia than anyone else. Dementia can affect *anyone*, regardless of race, culture, physical fitness, social and socioeconomic status, or intelligence.

# Misconception

*'Some people are so shrewd, they couldn't possibly be demented.'*

Many dementing people do show a surprising shrewdness. Those who are suspicious will probe and question what is said to them and are quick to pick up an untruth. Others show a surprising cunning, for example, the ability to calculate a complex way of 'escape' from home or nursing home by manipulating locks or finding their way out through a maze of corridors and buildings. Others are capable of deviousness, for example, the diabetic who obtains sweets and chocolates by persuading strangers to buy them for him or her.

# Misconception

*'Some of them try to make out they're worse than they really are, but they seem able to remember when it suits them.'*

One of the paradoxes of dementia is the up-and-down nature of the way some people act. Occasional good days bring flashes of understanding and memory that is so clear, and thinking that seems so logical, that the person seems normal. Unfortunately, these moments soon pass.

**People with dementia have adult needs and feelings.**
**Meet the needs. Respond to the feelings.**

# CHAPTER TWO

# About dementia

Dementia is a syndrome which describes a disorder of memory, thinking and behaviour.

Dementia is caused by a number of serious diseases that destroy brain cells.

Alzheimer's disease is the most common of these diseases.

Dementia can be thought of as brain failure.

Dementia worsens over time, progressing from a mild through to a moderate and finally to a severe stage.

Dementia progresses at different rates. One person may live for a number of years after diagnosis, another just a short time.

This handbook is about the more advanced stages of the disorder.

**Many treatable disorders can be mistaken for dementia. A correct diagnosis is essential.**

**Dementia** is a term used to describe a number of symptoms or characteristics caused by diseases which attack, damage and destroy brain tissue. These diseases seriously interfere with memory, thinking, judgment, speech, coordination and behaviour, and seriously affect the day-to-day functioning of the affected person.

# Dementia has many names

The word 'dementia' comes from two Latin words which mean 'away' and 'mind', and you will often hear a person with dementia referred to as 'losing their mind' or being 'out of their mind'. These phrases are very descriptive of the condition because it is the activity of the brain that we call the mind which is affected by the disease. Many other terms have been applied to dementia: organic brain syndrome, senility, pre-senile dementia, arteriosclerosis. Some of these names are still used, but now it is more usual to refer to the disease by name, for example Alzheimer's disease, Pick's disease, Lewy body disease; or simply 'dementia' or 'dementing illness'.

# Dementia and older age

Earlier this century dementia was considered to be a normal part of ageing, thus the term 'senile dementia'. We now know that this is not so; some very old people are unaffected by dementia, while much younger brains may show signs of one of the diseases.

In 1907, Dr Alois Alzheimer first described the disease which bears his name in a woman who was fifty-six years old. However, older people are more at risk of developing dementia, in the same way that there is more likelihood of arthritis, stroke, cancer and heart attack occurring in old age.

# The diseases

The most common of the dementia illnesses is Alzheimer's disease, which accounts for approximately sixty per cent of all cases diagnosed, followed by vascular dementia (multi-infarct and ischaemic) with an incidence of approximately fifteen to twenty per cent. Dementia can also result from a number of other diseases and conditions, some of which occur rarely.

Dementia disorders tend to fall into two loose groupings: those where the dementia is the main or *primary* disability; and those where the dementia is *secondary* to another illness, and may or may not occur with that disease.

Primary dementias include:
- dementia of the Alzheimer's type
- vascular dementia
- Lewy body disease
- fronto-temporal lobe dementia
- Pick's disease
- Creutzfeldt-Jakob disease
- Huntington's disease

Secondary dementia may occur with conditions such as:
- alcoholism
- brain injury
- brain tumour
- Parkinson's disease and other neurological disorders
- AIDS
- vitamin $B_{12}$ deficiency
- thyroid deficiency
- calcium excess
- syphilis

# Dementia-like symptoms

There are a number of medical conditions which have symptoms similar to those of a dementia illness and which can be mistaken for such. In particular, depression, which is common in older people, can have symptoms similar to those of a dementia illness and without a specialist diagnosis can be hard to distinguish from that disorder. Other disorders that fall into this category include effects of uncontrolled diabetes, prescription-drug misuse, heart and liver failure, urinary tract infection and other infections.

Whereas most true dementias are incurable, these conditions are treatable and potentially curable and to avoid misdiagnosis, it is essential that a medical/psychiatric consultation and psychological assessment be conducted.

# Rate of deterioration

Dementia is progressive and worsens over time. Symptoms are mild in the early stages. In the more advanced stages there is an increase in confusion and disorientation. Additional symptoms may develop and previous ones disappear.

In some of the literature you will find that between three and seven stages of Alzheimer's disease have been identified, each stage with a definite set of symptoms. However not all dementias will conform to this pattern, although most will progress from a mild through to moderate to a very severe stage. For some the disease runs its course from diagnosis to death over a number of years; for others the decline is rapid.

Deterioration during the course of dementia of the Alzheimer's type is gradual and insidious, whereas in the case of multi-infarct dementia the decline is step-like. If you are in daily contact with a person with Alzheimer's-type dementia the decline may almost go unnoticed, whereas with multi-infarct dementia you may observe immediate deterioration after each stroke or cerebro-vascular accident (CVA).

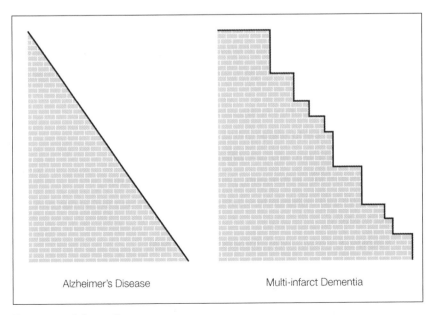

Alzheimer's Disease                    Multi-infarct Dementia

**Progress of dementia**

## MENTAL CAPACITIES THAT DECLINE WITH DEMENTIA

- recent memory
- immediate and distant memory
- capacity to use and understand words
- sense of where the body is in space, or where body parts are in relationship to objects and other people
- capacity to monitor the 'right' and 'wrong' of behaviour
- capacity to initiate or cease speech or activity
- comprehension of what is going on in the world around

## CHARACTERISTICS

When the capacities listed above are diminished or lost, a person will exhibit several of the following characteristics:

- cannot recall recent events;
- may not recall immediate or past events;
- is confused about:

    —time and place,

    —people, for example, mixes up mother/daughter, husband/father,

    —things—cannot name and misuses objects, for example, knife and fork

- is agitated and restless, walks aimlessly, seeks to escape, wanders away, clings and follows;
- has difficulty in initiating or stopping actions;
- has difficulty in performing routine tasks;
- misunderstands and misuses words;
- repeats questions, statements, actions and movements;
- sees, hears and believes things that are not happening (delusions and hallucinations);
- is suspicious (loses, hides, forgets and accuses);
- is demanding, noisy and aggressive;
- is apathetic, withdrawn and depressed;
- engages in disinhibited behaviour, for example, undressing in public places.

*Other changes*

Changes in personality and mood often take place and these may be due to a number of factors: changes in the brain, reaction to the environment, or psychiatric symptoms. Functioning may also be affected by physical disabilities such as impaired eyesight, hearing and mobility, or chronic illness, injury and incontinence.

## Individual differences

Not all dementing illnesses will have the same characteristics. The ways in which a person is affected will depend on the type of illness and the parts of the brain that are affected. With frontal lobe dementias, for instance, there is likely to be a tendency towards behavioural problems such as aggression but less effect on short-term memory loss. Also, there can be marked differences in symptoms or characteristics in the mild and moderate stages of the same illness. One person may retain the ability to do certain things or carry on a fairly normal life for quite a long time, while another needs considerable help even in the early stages of the disease. Eventually all will present with the same degree of disability.

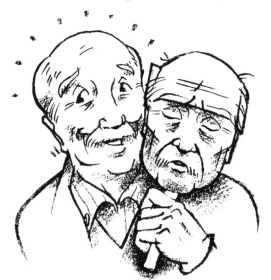

Discover the person behind the illness...

# CHAPTER THREE

# About the person with dementia

Throughout life we learn innumerable patterns of behaviour and movements which are stored in our minds, many of which we use without even thinking. Consider some of these patterns:

◆ language—thousands of words, and their use and how we communicate in speech and writing;
◆ recognition of people and their place in our lives;
◆ how to distinguish between objects, and their uses;
◆ domestic skills, such as cooking and sewing and gardening;
◆ self-care—such as bathing, teeth cleaning and dressing;
◆ work skills, such as typing, accounting, painting and driving;
◆ games—how to play them and their rules;
◆ appropriate behaviour in different situations;
◆ making judgments and decisions;
◆ developing ideas, being creative.

All this and much, much more is learned and stored in our minds and remembered. But when a person is affected by dementia these patterns gradually become distorted and are eventually lost. The affected person becomes confused and is handicapped in conducting his or her daily life.

A person in the more advanced stages of dementia will have several of the characteristics listed on page 14. Amongst the most commonly found are:

◆ memory loss
◆ confusion
◆ difficulty in understanding and using words
◆ inability to organise and coordinate thoughts, ideas, actions and movements
◆ delusions, hallucinations and confabulations
◆ excessive walking and wandering

# MEMORY LOSS

◆ Forgetting is temporary. Memory loss is permanent.
◆ Memory loss may be uneven, patches of memories may be retained.
◆ In many dementia illnesses, recent memories are lost first.
◆ An ability or part of a skill is often remembered.
◆ Memory can be gently prompted by:
  —using cues as triggers to stimulate memory;
  —using sight, smell, hearing, touch and taste.
◆ People gain pleasure when they remember.
◆ If trying to remember makes the person overanxious, stop prompting.

**Praise builds self-esteem.**

## HAGAR THE HORRIBLE                    by Dik Browne

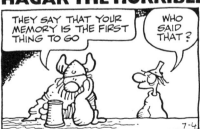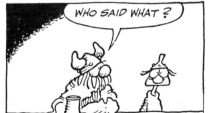

> Mrs Anderson greets the social worker each morning with a welcoming smile.
>
> 'Good morning. How nice to see you again. Do you live here? I know you, don't I? I've just forgotten your name.'
>
> 'I'm Julia, the social worker. I work here.'
>
> 'Of course, how silly of me, you're Julia, you're the social worker. Do you live here?'
>
> 'No. I live in my own house.'
>
> 'I've met you somewhere before. What is your name?'
>
> 'Julia.'
>
> 'Do you live here?'
>
> 'I live at home.'
>
> Mrs Anderson has no immediate memory. She forgets people and where they fit into her life, what she did or where she was the moment before.

# Memory loss and forgetting

Memory loss is permanent; forgetting is temporary. You might forget where you left your car keys, or where you left your car in the supermarket car park, or you may even forget someone's name. Everybody does this at some time or another. That is absent-mindedness or forgetting. On the other hand, if you think you still own a car you sold five years ago, or if you no longer remember that you are married, that is memory loss.

In most instances, people with dementia tend to have difficulty recalling recent and sometimes immediate past events. As the disease advances, long-term memory will also fade.

### *Not all memories are lost*

Memory differs from person to person. One person may be able to recollect a recent experience, while another will retain memories of some distant events until quite a late stage in the disease. Sometimes short-term memory stays remarkably intact.

> Dora remembers that her husband visited yesterday, her daughter is coming tomorrow and that her son lives in London. She reminds

the nurse of mealtimes or when it is time for a shower, but she does not know how to go to the dining room or turn on taps. Another person may not be able to remember exactly when an event occurred, but will know that it happened recently.

A person whose ability to communicate is impaired may well remember, but be unable to tell you. Because there are individual differences in remembering, it is important to pick up signs—facial expressions or body movement may evidence a flash of memory.

### *Significant experiences may be remembered*

The more significant the experience, the more likely it is to be remembered.

Helen remembers feeding the ducks in the park each week and Audrey often talks about climbing the tree in her grandparents' garden. Jack recalls that his daughter brought his briefcase recently.

Women residents in a Jewish dementia-specific unit, with little or no prompting, were able to carry out the ritual for preparation for the Sabbath, reminded only that it was Friday.

———

Five months after I had worked at a dementia unit, I met a group of the residents at a function. All except one spontaneously remembered me, although many of them no longer knew my name. On returning to the unit, some of them were able to relate the meeting to staff there.

### *A skill may be remembered*

Even when most memories are lost, a skill or part of a skill can be remembered.

William, once a concert pianist, is totally dependent on staff for his daily care. He doesn't recognise his family now, and cannot put words together or understand simple directions. Yet he frequently sits at the piano, opens the lid and plays a piece of classical music.

———

James, while the ability to pursue his trade as a watchmaker was long lost, could apply his skills to building mobiles and helping his grandchildren assemble Meccano pieces.

———

Mrs Jason became the self-appointed 'housewife' of the dementia unit and could be seen at all times of the day, vacuuming, sweeping and dusting.

# Prompting memory

You can prompt memory by talking about things, people and experiences that are familiar to the person with dementia. Recall recent pleasurable incidents and people who are significant in the dementing person's life. Give the person time, opportunity and encouragement to respond. Remembering can be an achievement, so praise or recognise in some way that achievement.

### *Using questions to prompt*

Questioning can often elicit a positive response from a person with dementia, leading to a pleasurable dialogue. However, we may be tempted to ask questions, often it seems for no better reason than to test their memories: 'Do you remember what you had for lunch?' 'Do you remember who came to see us this morning?' 'Do you remember this?' 'Do you remember that?'

This type of direct question may bring a blank or negative reaction. The question 'Where do you live?' created such anxiety in one lady, remembering the death of her husband, that it caused her to have a catastrophic reaction.

On the other hand, statements such as 'We went to the park in the bus this morning', or 'We had lunch in the garden today' or 'Your husband has a lovely smile' are likely to stimulate the person's memory and bring an interested response.

To use questions that require a simple 'yes' or 'no' answer can sometimes be inappropriate in prompting memory—the person, sensing that an answer is required, will often automatically respond with a 'yes' or a 'no' without meaning.

Also what can be forgotten is that even though a person may have dementia they are still entitled to privacy and they may be aware that their privacy is being invaded.

> They told me at the nursing home that Mrs Nicolic disliked swimming and refused to go on weekly swimming excursions.
>
> 'I hear you don't like swimming,' I remarked later, trying to make conversation.
>
> 'My business! My business!' she screamed at me, leaving me in no doubt about her deep resentment at my intrusion into her personal life.
>
> ———
>
> One usually gregarious man reacted to probing questions from staff by turning his back and maintaining a stony silence.

Before asking questions it is advisable to determine the purpose of the question. In the effort to reawaken memory are you attempting to:

- stimulate the person to socialise or interact with you?
- elicit necessary information?
- simply be curious?

### Using cues to prompt

A *cue* is an experience, person, anecdote or object that acts as a 'trigger' to stimulate the person to remember. The more familiar and the more significant a cue is to the person, the more likely it is to trigger memory. Use as many cues as possible to prompt memory. Photographs, flowers, magazines, pictures, posters, ornaments, films and music can all be used.

Talk to families and friends—they can provide you with information and objects that will act as cues.

### Using the senses as cues

We often underestimate the benefits of using the senses to stimulate memory: sight, smell, taste, touch and hearing can all be significant in prompting a memory. Music will often awaken a memory, as will a perfume, a smell or a colour. One woman talks about her travels whenever she hears a low-flying aircraft, while a man remembers his interest in car racing when passing vehicles accelerate loudly. For women, the colour, perfume, feel and look of make-up appeals to so many senses.

Just think how many senses an apple might stimulate: colour to be admired, fragrance to be smelled and a smooth and satiny surface to touch. You can taste its sweetness as you hear it crunch. It is surprising how many memories can be stimulated by an apple: climbing the tree as a child, walking through the orchard, making apple pie, a family gathering, or even the apples that a friend brought yesterday.

Do not overlook the benefits of exploiting the senses—there are many sensual experiences that will trigger memory.

### Why bother to prompt?

Judging by facial expression and other responses, people gain considerable satisfaction and pleasure when even the smallest memory returns. Where several people are sitting together, one person's recollection often leads to a trickle of memories from others. Self-esteem increases with the achievement of remembering and in response to encouragement and praise.

## The distress of memory loss

A person is sometimes aware of poor memory and may be distressed or even depressed by this. Prompting should be gentle, and if you notice signs of anxiety when the person is trying hard to remember, stop prompting. You might ask 'Can I help you remember?'. But before you prompt or contradict a mistaken memory, ask yourself 'What am I going to achieve?'. If you are unsure, or if the answer is 'nothing', stop.

If the person is aware of and expresses concern about memory loss, recognise that concern: 'You're upset because you can't remember', or 'It worries you when you forget'. A fading memory, together with other intellectual and emotional impairments, contributes to the person becoming confused and muddled in much of what they do.

# CONFUSION

The person who is confused often:

◆ fails to recognise and mixes up people, for example, mistakes son for father, nurse for mother, and so on;
◆ does not know where he or she is or cannot find his or her way around;
◆ is unable to measure how quickly or slowly time passes;
◆ does things at inappropriate times, for example, cooks breakfast at midnight;
◆ cannot name objects and uses tools incorrectly;
◆ suffers frustration and anxiety when aware of being confused.

---

**Recognise and respond to frustration and anxiety. Reassure the person. Stay with him or her.**

---

As the brain deteriorates, the person becomes more confused about what goes on around them. They may no longer be able to identify family or friends, or to recognise and correctly use everyday objects and tools. The dementing person becomes lost in time and space, not knowing where they are, and having no concept of time. When to sleep, when to wake and which meal follows which become a blur.

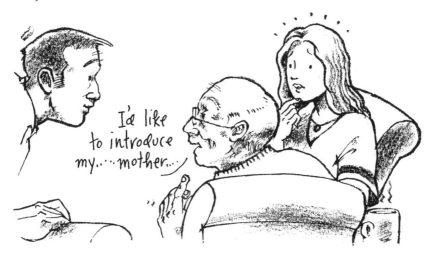

# Mixing up people

The dementing person may mix up or fail to identify people they have known well for a long time. This is one of the most difficult aspects for those close to them to deal with. It is upsetting to be mistaken for your grandmother or uncle; it is hard to understand why your loved one remembers you one day and not the next.

> Each afternoon, Mrs Jessup says to her husband, 'You'd better go now, my husband will be angry if he comes home and finds you here.'
>
> The only way he can pacify her is to go outside for a few minutes. On returning, she usually recognises and greets him as her husband.
>
> ———
>
> Miss Curry's brain has erased most of her adult life. She refers to staff and others around her as her mother, father, teacher, and so on.
>
> ———
>
> Mr Alanbee insists that one of the young residential care workers is his niece. He calls her by the niece's pet name, chats to her about 'shared' experiences and relatives, and attempts to cuddle and kiss her each time he sees her.

# Recognising a familiar face

Even though the dementing person may not be able to identify people or where they fit into their lives, they may recognise a visitor, for example. They may show pleasure either in words or actions when that person appears, often greeting them effusively.

# Confusing the place

> Mrs Terry does not recognise the house where she has lived for forty years. She frequently demands, 'I want to go home now', probably recalling her childhood home. She is reassured when the family does not try to explain, but says, 'We'll go soon.'
>
> ———

Ivy insists that the nursing home is in the country town where she lived twenty years ago. She is frustrated when the telephone numbers she dials fail to answer but is satisfied when the nurse suggests the phone might be out of order.

However, when anyone tries to convince her that this is the city and that her home is here now, she becomes argumentative and aggressive.

# Change increases confusion

Change to unfamiliar surroundings, even for a day, invariably increases the dementing person's confusion. Admission to hospital, respite care or a move to a nursing home where everyone is strange is frightening to someone who cannot comprehend.

Imagine how you would feel if you were lost in space!

## *Strong reactions to change*

Strong reactions to increasing fear and confusion about new surroundings are common. The person may wander, refuse to eat or cooperate with staff, become depressed, tearful, withdrawn, or verbally and physically aggressive. They may have difficulty in sleeping, wake during the night and, alone and lost, panic.

When the person receives your constant understanding and support and becomes used to the new surroundings they will invariably settle. The effects of change are also discussed in Chapters 8 and 9.

# Confusion about time

Just as the dementing person becomes lost in space, they may also become lost in time.

## *Time no longer exists*

In the advanced stages of dementing illness, time may no longer matter; it has ceased to exist.

## *Time cannot be measured*

Some dementing people are aware of time but cannot measure how slowly or quickly it passes. A few minutes seems like an hour, or everything happens 'yesterday' or 'a little while ago'. 'You've been gone a long time' is familiar to every carer who steps out of the room for a minute or two, just as 'You haven't been to see me for weeks' is to the family who visits daily.

> A woman whose husband visits on his way home from work paces up and down near the hostel gate. She comes inside when it is explained it will be hours yet before he comes. Five minutes later, she returns to the gate, to pace again. Not only may she have forgotten the explanation, but she cannot understand or measure time.

## *Anticipation*

The woman above who anticipates her husband's visit is probably worried she will miss him. It is not unusual for confusion, anticipation and anxiety to go hand-in-hand.

> About an hour after he arrives on his first day, the man at the day respite centre asks repeatedly 'When will my wife come?' or anxiously reassures himself 'My wife will be here soon'. He is feeling abandoned in a strange place and concerned that his wife will leave him there.
>
> ———
>
> The hostel resident who enjoys the weekly outing repeatedly asks 'How long before the bus trip?'

## *How do you answer?*

There is probably not much point in answering either by saying, for example, 'At one o'clock'. Someone who has no idea when one o'clock will be will only be further frustrated and anxious. They may understand better, or at least be satisfied for a while, if you associate time with a regular occurrence, for example:

- ◆ 'After you've had your lunch.'
- ◆ 'When you have had your tablets.'
- ◆ 'You need to have a rest first.'

Sometimes words like 'soon' and 'afterwards' said in a reassuring tone will be enough, but be prepared for the query 'When is soon/afterwards?'

## The right thing at the wrong time

> Some mornings Dorothy gets up at two o'clock and prepares breakfast for her husband.
>
> ———
>
> James phones his daughter several times between midnight and 4 am, just to have a chat.
>
> ———
>
> At 6 am Emily dresses and orders a taxi to take her to a 3 pm dental appointment.
>
> ———
>
> Alf waits at the door of his unit for the day-care bus at ten o'clock at night.

These people all know what it is they want to do and how to do it, but they have no idea of the appropriate time.

## Clocks

Clocks do not seem to lessen confusion about time. However, some people do gain a sense of achievement from 'reading' the time, even though they do not know what it means. To encourage this, place clocks with large figures where they can be easily seen.

# Confusion about objects

> Mr Jones picks up the soap and seems puzzled. He carefully examines it, turns it over, squeezes it, smells it and finally, deciding it is a cake or scone, takes a bite.
>
> ———
>
> Mrs Paterson sets fire to her kitchen when she tries to cook vegetables in a plastic bowl.

Confusion about objects leads to many seemingly strange behaviours: washing the floor with the best lace tablecloth, or pouring orange juice into a plate of hot soup. Gently redirecting the person's movements each time the object or tool is misused is often effective, although it is unlikely to be remembered.

Only rarely does someone use an object dangerously, and then often only as a result of provocation. If the person is known to be aggressive, remove an object that is likely to be used as a weapon.

# Frustration and anxiety

The person who realises they are confused may at times be frustrated and highly anxious or even become depressed. If they cannot express frustration in words, you may be able to pick up the feelings from facial expression or actions.

### *Recognise, respond, reassure*

It comforts the person for you to recognise these feelings.

- Respond to the feeling: 'You're frightened because you don't know where you are.'
- If the person is able to verbalise their feelings, encourage this.
- Reassure:
  —'You're safe, you are at…'
  —'You're a bit mixed up about the time? I'll remind you when it's time to go.'
  —'You're worried your wife will forget you? Don't worry, she'll be here when you've had afternoon tea.'

If you are repeatedly reassuring, anxiety will lessen in most instances. They may not know who you are or where you fit into their life, but you are a familiar face and they know you care.

### *Provide company*

Try sitting for a while with an anxious person; hold their hand. Walking with them can also be an effective way to lessen anxiety.

Stay with the anxious person until they settle. If the anxiety or depression persists, seek professional advice.

# Full-time care is needed

By the time a person has developed a severe degree of confusion, short-term memory is also usually seriously impaired. This person is at risk. If there is not a full-time carer, hostel or nursing-home care should be considered.

# MISUNDERSTANDING AND MISUSING WORDS*

- When the parts of the brain that control the use of words and comprehension are affected, the person with dementia will gradually lose the ability to talk in a way that you can understand. The mind cannot find the right words or string them together in a way that makes sense.
- There will be difficulty:
  —understanding what you are telling or asking (ears may be hearing, but the mind cannot grasp the meaning of the words);
  —writing a message or even a name, or understanding what it is that he or she is reading (even though the words may be recognised, the brain cannot comprehend their meaning).
- The person experiencing word difficulties:
  —may have a limited vocabulary; or substitute, explain or describe a lost word;
  —may use nonsense words, mix up ideas or have unintelligible speech;
  —may gradually revert to a native language but make no sense in any language;
  —may experience extreme frustration and become angry.

---

**Paradox: A person who cannot comprehend the meaning of written words often understands signs such as 'Exit' and is able to follow arrows.**

---

*Guidelines for communicating are discussed in Chapter 8, especially on p.157.

Many people with dementia have great difficulty carrying on a conversation and expressing ideas. Even asking a rational question or communicating their needs seem to be impossible.

As well as difficulties associated with the dementia, other factors must be taken into account to give a complete picture. For example, a stroke may deprive the person of speech so that they are no longer able to talk, and a hearing impairment may make it extremely difficult to hear what is being said. Words that follow each other too quickly or a speaker's voice too low will make hearing difficult. Someone with poor eyesight may not be able to detect a speaker who is too far away and will not know who the person is talking to.

# Two major problems

You will frequently encounter two major problems when trying to talk with a person with dementia. One is the inability to tell you something in a way that makes sense, even though she or he is still able to talk. The other is difficulty in comprehending what you are saying or in understanding what it is that she or he is reading.

There are special parts of the brain that control our use of words and our comprehension. When these parts are damaged the person will not be able either to find the right word to use or to string words together so that they make sense. There will be great difficulty in understanding what people are saying, and sometimes there will be no understanding at all. Also there may be an inability to write a sensible message, and even though the person may recognise the words that he or she is reading, they may not comprehend the meaning of the words.

# Misunderstanding words

The problem experienced in understanding words is sometimes called 'word deafness' and 'word blindness'. This is because the person's eyes can still see and ears can still hear. It is the mind that cannot grasp the meaning of the words.

## *The spoken word*

In the more advanced stages of dementia, there can be great difficulty in understanding what people are saying.

> Staff in the hostel believe Mrs Penny is uncooperative. When the nurse says 'Come here please', she replies 'Yes' but remains seated. When asked 'Would you like a cup of tea?', she smiles and says 'Yes' but makes no attempt to fetch it.

Mrs Penny is not uncooperative. She does not understand the words. Like many who do not comprehend, Mrs Penny automatically answers 'Yes' or 'No' to every request.

## *The written word*

It is not unusual for people with dementia to be able to read and understand signs. Others will appear to read magazines and newspapers but not comprehend the meaning.

> Every morning, Mrs Brown 'reads' her newspaper from cover to cover, just as she has done all her adult life. When asked, she willingly reads aloud a headline or a sentence, but she cannot explain its meaning.

On the other hand:

> Mr Opit, who can no longer talk, seems to understand what he is reading, judging by his facial expression and occasional laughter as he browses through the magazines his daughter brings.

# Misusing words

> Mrs Roberts approaches a visitor and confides, 'You know the girls? ... music and thing ... you know, garplop ... didn't tell me about ... shopping ... worried ... shoes must prippy.' She speaks rapidly, misusing and making up words. She cannot complete sentences nor express her thoughts or complete ideas.

The noises Mrs Timson makes through clenched teeth do not sound much like words, but she seems to be telling us something.

Mr Sharp holds a pen and his hand makes writing movements, but when he writes his name it looks like this:

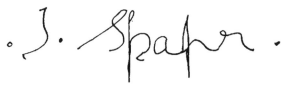

Even though the voice and hands are still working, these people have great difficulty in using words. They lack intelligible speech and cannot make written sense.

# Word problems

## Substituting

Substitution of a word that has a similar meaning to or sounds like the right word is common.

'I want to go into the flowers.' [garden]
'Please pass my kitten.' [knitting]
'They went ... in there ... through the hole.' [doorway]

## Explaining

When someone describes or explains the function of the lost word, the meaning is fairly easily understood.

♦ 'My son brought me a ... a stick ... sharp you put in ink ... on paper.' [pen]
♦ 'We had a lovely time at the ... out of the bus ... walked ... trees ... pond with ducks ... had our lunch.' [visit to the park]

## Limited vocabulary

The richness of speech is significantly impaired and the number of words the person has available is greatly reduced. Words may still be used correctly, but sentences are often short or single words only are used: 'Toilet'; 'A cigarette?'; 'Hungry'; or 'Go out now'.

### Nonsense words

The meaning of this sort of dialogue is usually very difficult to understand. The words seem to be made up; sometimes a combination of unrelated syllables or incomplete words are used.

### Garbled sentences

In the anecdote on page 31, Mrs Roberts has a typical garbled sentence pattern. She strings words together in scraps of sentences, her thoughts are mixed up, she jumps from one idea to another and she uses nonsense words. It is almost impossible to understand what she is trying to communicate.

### Pressure of speech

When speech is pressured, the person speaks rapidly, hardly drawing breath between words and sentences or sounds and it can be almost impossible to interrupt. Pressured speech often accompanies a garbled sentence pattern and babbling.

### Babbling

The person makes a series of short sounds, a little like a child learning to talk. Babbling often gives way to grunts and noises.

## Less serious word problems

Problems with words are not always as serious as those discussed above. People may simply 'lose' a word, hesitate overlong before stringing words together, or use short sentences to make themselves understood. Speech may also be affected when a person is anxious or unwell.

## English as a second language

Even though people from non-English-speaking backgrounds may have been fluent in the English language, it is likely that they will revert to their first language as the disease progresses. It is quite common for a mixture of the first and acquired languages to be used. Trying to translate for these people may be of little help because the understanding and use of words in the native tongue will also decline rapidly, and the person may not make sense in, or understand, any language.

However, even where there is little understanding, a person may be overjoyed to hear their native tongue spoken.

## Frustration

People with word difficulties may suffer intense frustration and anxiety at their inability to communicate clearly. They may know what it is that they want to say or tell you that they have understood you, but be unable to do either. They may react with tears or anger.

## Return of an earlier speech pattern

Sometimes a person will revert to an earlier, and what was for them a more normal speech pattern. The babbler may utter single intelligible words, the Italian speaker may ask a question in English. Mrs Roberts (above) occasionally reverts to a short, sensible sentence.

# DIFFICULTY IN COORDINATING THOUGHTS AND ACTIONS

The person with dementia may know what she or he wants to do, but the failing brain cannot transpose the ideas or thoughts into actions.

The brain gradually ceases to organise, coordinate and monitor movements and actions.

Difficulties range from the inability to perform a single movement, such as lifting a hand, to not being able to accomplish a whole task, such as dressing. The sequence of movements for sitting, standing and walking is often lost.

Sometimes an action can be accomplished if you help the person to start the movement.

Encourage independence, but do not expect more than the person is capable of doing.

**Some people can learn simple tasks and new patterns of behaviour, but generally new learning is fraught with difficulty or not possible in the more advanced stages of the diseases.**

# Coordination

Have you ever counted the number of single movements you make to dress each morning?

◆ You put on several pieces of clothing where each piece fits.
◆ Your body and limbs move so that you can pull on, up, over, through.
◆ Your fingers make fine movements to tie, zip up, button-up, hook-up.
◆ You notice you have odd shoes and you select those that match.

All this you accomplish more or less without thinking. Your brain automatically organises and coordinates the movements for each action and directs the sequence in which you put on the garments. It monitors what you have done and signals that red shoes do not go with the orange dress. Or that the patterned tie looks better than the plain blue one.

You would not put your singlet on over your cardigan! Yet this is what a person with dementia might do when the mind has lost the ability to organise, coordinate and monitor their actions.

# Impaired coordination

Impaired coordination affects the carrying out of whole tasks or activities, such as washing-up and playing cards, or simple actions, such as lifting the hand to scratch an itchy nose. Even though someone may know what she or he wants to do, they lack the ability to transpose those thoughts or wishes into actions. For example, a man may want to watch television but the message from the brain to press the button to turn on the power has been lost. Even simple tasks like cleaning teeth can be influenced, the message 'put the toothpaste on the brush, now lift the brush to your teeth, and brush' does not get through.

> Mrs Jones no longer knows the order for putting on her clothes, yet she won a needlework competition for nursing-home residents in her area.

## *How to get started*

Sometimes a person knows what to do but the capacity to begin a task or start a movement is lost. It is often considered that this person is lazy or lacks motivation but this is usually not so. She or he just cannot get started, in other words cannot *initiate* the action.

Earlier, we talked about Dora, who knew when it was time to shower but was not able to work the taps. She was hungry and wanted to eat, but she could not move towards the dining room without direction.

One way to assist a person to get started is to use a cue. Gently prompting the first movement acts as a cue which 'triggers' the action or task. Don't be discouraged if the cue does not work the first time; you may have to repeat the same cue several times. On the other hand, you may have to try several different cues before you find one that works.

> Although hungry, Keith sits gazing at his plate, not responding to 'Eat your dinner, Keith'. He becomes interested in his dinner when the spoon is placed in his hand, but still does not eat. Only when his hand is guided to his mouth, does he start feeding himself.
>
> Without this prompting he cannot start the movement, becomes highly agitated and wanders off.
>
> ───────
>
> Imagine a room. People are sitting on chairs placed around the walls. They stare at the floor, at the walls, at each other, not noticing staff move around or the occasional visitor come and go. One woman leaves her chair, wanders aimlessly for a few minutes, and returns to sit again. Another gets up and wanders off.
>
> Two volunteers arrive. They use several cues to start the activity. The music and words of old songs wafting from the portable cassette player awaken memories. The volunteers move among the group, prompting, starting movements, singing, swaying, guiding a hand to move in time with the rhythm, encouraging.

Heads rise, eyes slowly come alive as the sitters join in, hands tapping and feet moving to the rhythm of the music. Some get up to dance.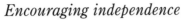

## Encouraging independence

Encourage the person to be independent for as long as it is possible for them to be.

It often seems quicker and less of a nuisance to do things for people: shower, dress, feed, fetch, carry, pick up. Or we may be moved to do these things because we care. To do things for people unnecessarily, however, deprives them of the satisfaction that comes from carrying out a task, either alone or with your help. There can be a sense of achievement even from combing hair or putting on a shoe independently. Sincere praise from the person supervising adds to feelings of self-esteem: 'You did well. You put the shoe on your foot. Good.'

If someone cannot accomplish a task alone, either ask if you can help or encourage them to assist you: 'Would you like to help me put these flowers in water?' or 'Would you help me put your clothes away?'

## Expecting too much causes frustration

There is a fine line between maintaining the dementing person's independence and expecting more than an individual is capable of accomplishing. We are often tempted to ask too much, especially of someone who still has some conversational skills, some comprehension and interacts well with others. This can be a social veneer or a front, which many people with dementia retain.

Do not expect the person to attempt a task that is too difficult for him or her. If after a few minutes of prompting, starting and encouraging, the movement or activity cannot be performed, *stop*. Insistence may result in frustration, confirms feelings of failure, and the consequence may be that impatience, distress and aggression may result. Or the person may 'switch off' or walk away.

Walking frames and quad sticks can help with sitting, standing and walking, although by the time this type of aid is needed, the person may have lost the ability to learn the movements necessary for their use. The wheeled type of frame is preferable, for with it the person does not have to coordinate lifting and placing the frame, as is necessary with other types.

Where there is the complication of a physical condition such as Parkinson's disease, an assessment by a physiotherapist or occupational therapist is advisable. A series of movements designed to help that person can then be prescribed.

### Encouragement and reassurance

Talk to the person, encourage and reassure them that they are safe. Explain each step before you attempt it and while it is being done.

**Encourage. Reassure. Praise.**

# DELUSIONS, HALLUCINATIONS AND CONFABULATION

Delusions are false ideas or beliefs; hallucinations are false sensations. Both are often bizarre and unbelievable.

Sometimes the delusion is associated with feelings of persecution and the person becomes extremely suspicious.

Delusions and hallucinations are often frightening.

Arguing and explanation will not convince the person that what they believe, see or hear is not happening. Treat it as real.

Confabulation is a story that is fabricated to fill in a gap in memory.

Confabulation is believed by the teller and is believable to the listener.

Before dismissing something as a delusion, hallucination or confabulation, check it out. It may be true.

It is not unusual for people with dementia to experience delusions and hallucinations. It is not certain whether these are the consequence of the dementia or whether there is another reason, such as a psychiatric disturbance. In some instances, these symptoms can be enhanced by prescription drugs.

## Delusions

A **delusion** is a false idea or belief. Delusions are unreal and can be strange and often bizarre. A person who is deluded has no control over their thoughts and is not telling lies. The experience or the ideas they are having are to them very real.

> A 75-year-old lady is convinced that her mother who died thirty years ago is still alive. She tells staff of the hostel where she lives, 'My mum is coming to take me to the pictures today', or 'I have to tidy the room ready for my mum, she is coming to stay with me for a few days'.

# Medication

When delusions and hallucinations persist, it is advisable to seek a consultation with a psychogeriatrician for a proper assessment. Delusions and hallucinations often respond to medication.

# Confabulation

People with dementia will often confabulate. It seems that, struggling to understand and make sense of a confused world, the person fabricates an explanation to fill in a gap in memory.

Unlike delusions and hallucinations, a confabulation is invariably associated with a real incident. Other differences are that confabulations:

- have a ring of truth;
- are fully believed by the teller;
- are equally believable to the listener;
- are seldom accompanied by anxiety.

### *Answering questions*

The person who confabulates will usually have ready answers to questions. For example:

*Question*: What did you have for breakfast?
*Confabulation*: Grilled tomato, cornflakes and toast.
*Fact*: Porridge, eggs, toast and marmalade.

### *Explaining what is not understood*

A husband or wife who is sick, overseas or working is a common confabulation among residents of nursing homes and hostels.

> A widower explains away the reason he is in the nursing home: 'My wife is sick and can't take care of me at home for a while. She might have to go to hospital, you know.'
>
> ———
>
> In a large hotel-like hostel, Janet and Mavis happily tell everyone: 'We've been coming here for holidays all of our lives'—even though the hostel has recently been built and they have only just met.

## *Not an excuse*

The woman who says 'I sat on a wet chair' when she loses bladder control is not making excuses. She is explaining what she believes happened and is reassured when the nurse says: 'Oh dear, that's uncomfortable. Let's go and put on some clean knickers.'

## *Modifying an unhappy situation*

On the rare occasion when the confabulation has the potential to concern the person, you can mostly prevent this by changing the situation.

> Mrs Jackson does not understand why her husband chats to 'that woman' (the supervisor) when he visits. She complains to everyone that they are having an affair. When he stops talking to staff in her presence, she stops complaining.

## *Consequences of confabulation*

Due to the nature of confabulation, the consequences can be more serious and more difficult to deal with than either a delusion or a hallucination.

> Mrs X had long been a favourite of the day-centre supervisor. One day she complained that her son had taken all her money. The supervisor at first put Mrs X's story down to confusion until she turned up one day with her bank book showing a recent withdrawal of a large sum of money. On questioning, Mrs X explained that her son had stolen the money and gone on a holiday to Europe. Mrs X's temporary carer could not throw any light on the matter and when the son returned from his business trip he was confronted by police.
>
> What was the true story? The son (who held his mother's enduring power of attorney) had withdrawn the money and invested it at a higher rate of interest than it was attracting in her bank account, as he usually did. He had explained this to his mother who, forgetting and finding the money had gone, fabricated the story to fill in the gap in her memory.

**People who wander away invariably become lost and must be accommodated in secure areas with ample walking space.**

**Sometimes undesirable walking can be modified by identifying the underlying reason.**

**It is essential to provide people with dementia with:**
**—ample space for walking;**
**—regular daily exercise;**
**—sufficient activity to prevent boredom;**
**—a calm environment.**

# Walking patterns

For many people with dementia, walking for exercise has been a normal part of life. Some continue their lifelong habit of walking for pleasure; some who lack sufficient physical activity because of confinement will walk for exercise. Others are agitated and restless, and pace frantically as though driven by extreme anxiety. Some just wander. They aimlessly stroll from room to room or around the garden. There are also those who have no idea of where they are or where they are going, and they need to be prevented from wandering away and putting themselves at risk of becoming lost or injured.

# People who like to walk

While it is essential to protect people from wandering away, we often regard all active walkers as 'wanderers' and restrict them in the same way as we restrict people who are at risk of wandering away and becoming lost. In fact, many people with dementia have a well-preserved sense of location. They can recognise where they are, can find their way around, and get considerable pleasure from walking. Mr Jakep, for example, knows exactly where he is:

His wife would lock him in the house to prevent him from wandering away if she had to go out. One day she returned home to find him reading the morning paper. Knowing they did not have the paper delivered, she asked him where he had found it. 'Oh,' he said, 'I just

> got out through the window and went up to the paper shop, then I came home and climbed back through the window again.'

To restrict or restrain such people from walking reduces the quality of their lives, causes frustration, anger and sometimes violent reactions.

> When Stella is diagnosed as suffering from Alzheimer's disease, the nursing home discontinues her regular walk, confining her to one section. She refuses to eat and has frequent angry outbursts until she is allowed to resume her daily rambles.

### *Make sure the person knows the way*

To assess whether it is safe to allow the person to walk alone, accompany them along the route and if, after a few times, you are satisfied that they are able to find the way home, a period of unrestricted walking each day could be allowed, even encouraged. Assess the person's sense of direction and location at least every two weeks.

## The excessive walker

Another type of walker is the restless person who walks incessantly. As mentioned before, sometimes this is as a result of insufficient exercise, particularly if the person is physically fit or has indulged in a lifetime of exercise or sport.

Excessive walking may also take the form of frantic pacing, the person appearing to be stressed and driven by anxiety. This anxiety is often triggered by an emotional reaction to something in the environment or a recollection from the past that has upset them. With others there does not seem to be a reason for the agitation. With agitated walking if you can identify the trigger for the behaviour, you may be able to lessen or prevent it.

> Mr Fetteren spent many years during World War II as a prisoner of war, often in solitary confinement. Now he suffers from Alzheimer's disease and is accommodated in a locked unit. He undoubtedly thinks he is back in the camp. He paces endlessly, frantically trying to escape.

> When he is taken outside the unit, his anxiety lessens and he sits quietly.

# Wandering and wandering away

The person who wanders has no control over this type of behaviour. It is probably due to a number of underlying causes, including confusion about location and seriously impaired memory. Fear, bewilderment or an anxiety-provoking incident may also contribute to the behaviour.

## *Two types of wanderers*

There are two types of wanderers. The first never attempts to leave familiar surroundings and will stroll endlessly and often happily in the immediate vicinity of where they live. This type of wanderer is not at risk but needs to be supervised as there is always the chance that one day they will go further afield.

The second type is the wanderer who will suddenly 'take off' and roam without heed to time or place. They do not seem to tire and are often found hours later, sometimes wet and cold, still walking kilometres from home. This type of wanderer will seldom, if ever, backtrack to their starting point, and will frequently become lost and sometimes injured.

It is difficult to understand why a person takes it into his or her head to wander away. Some seem just to begin to walk and then keep on walking. Others seem to have a definite idea of where they want to go, often to search for a friend from long ago or a childhood place that does not exist anymore.

> Mrs Ryan slips undetected through the hostel security gate and makes her way to the main road. She hails a taxi, giving the address of her childhood home, which was demolished years ago.
>
> ———
>
> Peter South catches the bus and train to the suburb where his daughter used to live, but on arrival he does not know where he is or why he came.

# Effects of strange surroundings

A move to new surroundings, even for a day, often triggers restlessness, incessant walking, pacing and wandering. If the person stays overnight in strange surroundings, they may become frightened when they waken and fail to recognise where they are and they may begin to wander. As the person becomes accustomed to the environment, however, anxiety will lessen and the stress-driven walking or wandering may ease or disappear.

# Security and supervision

The person who is at risk of wandering away must be accommodated in an enclosed and secure unit with plenty of space to ramble. But this is not enough for some. The competent 'escapologist' who is able to manipulate locks or jump fences, or the resident who slips out with someone else's visitors, requires continuous supervision. Regular head-counts at mealtimes are also a good idea.

To further reduce the risk, door alarms, electronic locks, tracking devices and other devices should be considered.

### *Identity bracelets*

For added protection, people at risk should wear an identity bracelet at all times. Where the person lives at home and repeatedly wanders away, the local police will often agree to the family providing them with a description and photograph for identification purposes.

# Modifying the behaviour

You can sometimes modify the person's excessive walking or wandering by:

◆ holding a hand or arm gently and walking alongside;
◆ talking quietly and soothingly;
◆ taking the person for a walk outside, first making sure they are not frightened by another unfamiliar place.

### *Providing diversions*

Rest points or other diversions to break up walking areas may distract the person who walks continuously or has a tendency to wander. Suggestions are:

- a seat at the end of the garden path and small tools with which to dig;
- birds in a secure aviary (this can attract attention for quite long periods);
- chairs and tables with books or articles to handle;
- easily accessible television (turned on);
- expendable craft material.

## Imposing limits on walking

As long as the person appears to gain satisfaction from walking and no physical and emotional stress is apparent, walking should not be limited. However, there are times when it is necessary to curtail walking.

For instance, physical exhaustion may result from continuous walking, feet and ankles may swell and feet may become rubbed and painful. Highly agitated walkers or those who follow and cling can upset others and so create management difficulties.

Encouraging the person to join activities such as craft, cooking, singing or watching television and so on will often keep him or her off their feet for a while. But in extreme cases, however, such as the need to prevent foot infection or injury, he or she may have to be physically restrained for a short time in order to prevent injury or infection as a result of the walking. Restraint by tying someone to a chair or bed is always undesirable and should only be used as a last resort, and then only after discussion with the person's doctor and family.

---

**A calm atmosphere, sufficient activity to prevent boredom and regular daily exercise reduce agitation.**

# CHAPTER FOUR

# Personality and mood changes and emotional reactions

Our abilities to think, remember, comprehend, concentrate, use language, make logical judgments, have ideas, and so on are called *cognitive abilities,* or *cognition.* When a person has dementia, cognitive abilities are always impaired.

The way we present to the world through our personalities, our mood and our emotions is called *affect* or *affective behaviour.* The person with dementia invariably undergoes changes in affect. In this chapter, we consider those changes.

## CHANGES IN PERSONALITY

There can be changes in personality as the disease progresses, although some people do retain their basic personalities.

Changes happen slowly and subtly, and often go unnoticed in the early stages.

Families and friends have difficulty relating to the changed person.

In some instances, all inhibitions are lost; some dementing people behave in ways that they would never, under any circumstances, have acted before.

The personality may undergo marked changes as the disease progresses so that it is difficult to recognise someone as the person they once were.

# Exaggeration of normal personality

In some instances the change takes the form of an exaggeration of the normal personality.

Suspicious people will become increasingly so and believe that they are being persecuted. The previously timid person may live in a continual state of fear; the woman who had a caring and affectionate nature may now kiss and cuddle indiscriminately or gently 'love' everyone.

# Personality reversal

Sometimes it seems that the personality becomes the opposite of the outward self before the dementia. The hitherto trusting person becomes suspicious; the gentle person becomes irritable and angry; and the calm person will have frequent outbursts of temper.

# Difficulty in relating

In the early stages of the disease small changes in the person's nature tend to go unnoticed, particularly by someone who is seeing them daily. But in the advanced stages the changes in personality may have become so marked that family and friends often do not know how to relate to the changed person.

> Mary and John are in their middle sixties. Mary notices John is not as gentle as he used to be. Because he has difficulty with words, he is frustrated. Breaking off in the middle of sentences, he reacts angrily towards Mary, accusing her of not listening or not believing. As his illness progresses, he sometimes storms out of the house, shouting abuse.
>
> Mary finds it hard to believe his changed personality is due to brain failure, pointing out that sometimes he is the old gentle,

reliable John. Even when he becomes suspicious and angry most of the time, she alternates between asking his advice as she has always done, and becoming distraught at his aggression.

## Disinhibited behaviour

Family and friends also find it difficult to tolerate behaviour that is out of social control—when the mind ceases to distinguish between the 'right' and 'wrong' of the way the person acts. The resultant change in personality is one that family and friends find it difficult to tolerate. The person loses control and behaves in a way that would have been unthinkable before. Such a person may loudly interrupt, complain noisily, hit and scratch, or undress in public. Uncharacteristic swearing, abusiveness and sexual misdemeanours are also consequences of the brain's failure to monitor behaviour.

Because of these extreme personality changes, you will often hear a carer say that the person with dementia is 'unrecognisable' as the person they used to be because of the marked change in his or her personality.

# LISTLESSNESS AND DEPRESSION

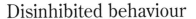

As dementia worsens, some people lose the ability to initiate activity and conversation and have difficulty in relating to others.

Because the person is indifferent and does not resist or argue, listlessness is sometimes mistaken for cooperation.

If listlessness is ignored, the person can become isolated and vacant. Involve the person in conversation and activities.

Listlessness may be a sign of depression.

Depression must be assessed, as it may:

—be due to some personal problem or environmental factor that can be modified;

—have a physical or biological cause and treatment with medication might be necessary.

# Listlessness

'I don't believe they have dementia, they're not like the dementing people I know. The patients in my nursing home are so sluggish,' remarked the nurse as she watched a video of a group of people actively engaged in a word game. 'My people just sit and do nothing, or wander around all day.'

In that nursing home, the belief was that listlessness and apathy were an inevitable consequence of the disease. No attempt was made to provide any sort of stimulation for their dementia residents, consequently even those who otherwise would have been interested assumed an air of dejection.

The person with dementia may lose the ability to start an activity or a conversation and have difficulty in relating to others. Inactivity and indifference can often be symptomatic of dementia but this is not always the case. There may be other reasons for a person's apathy and these should not be overlooked. She or he may be:

◆ ill
◆ bored
◆ unable to initiate activity
◆ emotionally upset
◆ depressed

## *Do not ignore listless behaviour*

The person who is quiet and withdrawn poses no problem for caregivers. The listless, apathetic one will seldom argue or resist direction, and is often regarded as being passively cooperative and 'a good patient' and is left to his or her own devices.

Whatever the reason, it is highly unlikely that the person is able to control listlessness, or change the apathetic mood without help, and it may persist long after the reason for it has passed. Left to his or her own devices the listless one will become increasingly dejected, isolated, staring vacantly into space, and may sink prematurely into oblivion. Do not let this happen!

## *Combating listless behaviour*

As we saw above listlessness is often dismissed as being inevitable and unchangeable. This is not so. In trying to combat apathy, you may find in the beginning that you have to pay the person a considerable amount of attention for little result. But gradually, as they respond to your interest and encouragement, they will improve.

You might find the following guidelines helpful in bringing about improvement in the person:

◆ Do not ignore them.
◆ Do not leave them sitting alone or on the fringe of the group.
◆ Involve them in activities.
◆ Converse about familiar topics or about what is happening in the environment at that moment.
◆ Include them in outings.
◆ If the person is chairbound, make sure he or she is not left alone.

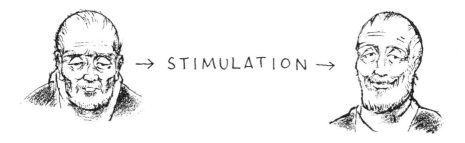

→ STIMULATION →

❝ The students are working in a ward of men with dementia. Their first exercise is to make 'contact' with any one patient. By mischance, one student chooses a man who has not been heard to speak for at least twelve months and spends his waking hours gazing into nothingness. After thirty minutes of her talking, prompting and smiling encouragement, he still does not respond. 'I did as you suggested and asked him "What would make you happy?" but I don't think he even understood me,' she despaired.

> Yet the student persisted, and a few days later she chirpily reported to me: 'That patient came up to me today. He took me by the hand, led me out to the verandah and pointed to the swallows nesting under the eaves. He said "Happy" and his eyes shone.'
>
> After a few months of the student's interest, the patient was encouraged to join the exercise sessions and is a member of the daily gardening group. More animated now, he enjoys 'chatting', even though he can only manage single words.

# Listlessness and depression

Listlessness can be a sign of depression. Where the person is thought to be suffering from depression, a psychiatric assessment is essential so that the correct treatment can be prescribed.

# Types of depression

### Changes in the brain

It is quite common for depression to be caused by changes in the brain that are associated with a disease.

### Psychiatric illness

The person's depressed state may be due to a mental illness. The person's melancholy mood will appear and worsen for no apparent reason.

### Reactive depression

We often refer to this as 'feeling depressed' or 'feeling miserable'. This form of depression is a 'normal' reaction to a distressing incident such as a death or a breakdown in a relationship. As with everyone, people with dementia will often suffer such depressions and it is not unusual for someone to be saddened by the deterioration associated with the illness. Another may not be able to cope with an incident that is causing unhappiness. Each feels helpless and may react by becoming withdrawn and despondent.

# Medication

In some forms of depression, treatment with appropriate medication brings about dramatic changes in the person's mood and energy and a renewed interest in life.

## *When medication helps*

Aware of his loss of memory and decreasing ability to make decisions, and fearful of becoming lost, Mr Pittie becomes withdrawn and despondent, often bursting into tears for no apparent reason. When family and friends visit the house, he retreats to his room or sits impassively. One day he attempts suicide by cutting his wrist and his wife asks for him to be referred to a psychiatrist. Antidepressant medication is prescribed.

Mr Pittie no longer dwells on his advancing Alzheimer's disease, his interest in reading returns and he is more inclined to become involved in what goes on around him.

## *When medication does not cure*

When someone suffers from a reactive depression, modifying the reason for the depression will often bring about a change in mood. There are times, however, when the reason cannot be changed and we have to help the person adjust to the situation.

Depression is a common reaction when the person moves to a nursing home or hostel. Medication may temporarily ease the pain, but eventually the person needs to deal with the changes in his life. If you can encourage them to express their feelings and let them know you understand, no matter how long it takes, this will add to the effectiveness of medication.

Miss Wisp is transferred from the hostel to a dementia unit for 'her own protection'. No longer permitted to call a taxi to visit her many friends or to stroll to the local shopping centre and TAB to place her bets, she becomes despondent. She complains, 'I wish I could die.' She seldom leaves her room, eats little and sleeps fitfully.

She is transferred to a psychiatric hospital where she is treated for depression, but on returning to the dementia unit and the same restrictive lifestyle, she again becomes dejected. A companion is employed to take her out for a few hours each day. She brightens up and antidepressants are no longer necessary. Hospital treatment may have been avoided if someone had thought to take this or a similar step earlier.

---

**Antidepressants must be prescribed cautiously as they may have undesirable side effects.**

---

# EMOTIONAL REACTIONS

---

**Do not discourage expression of feelings.**

**As the brain fails, expression of feelings may become inappropriate, shallow, extreme or out of proportion to the situation.**

**Extreme emotional reactions are often triggered by the person's feelings of anxiety and helplessness, the reason for which may not be immediately apparent.**

**Some extreme emotional reactions are quiet and often overlooked.**

**Catastrophic reactions can often be avoided.**

**Unless the situation causing the reaction is modified, episodes may become more frequent and more intense.**

**While the person may not be able to indicate what triggered an emotional reaction, you—by observing closely—may be able to identify and rectify the reason and prevent a recurrence.**

**A calm, caring environment helps to prevent extreme emotional reactions.**

---

People with dementia experience a range of normal emotions, including anger and grief, and express their feelings appropriately. This should be encouraged rather than discouraged.

As the brain fails, however, the person may not comprehend what is going on around him or her and become confused, deluded, suspicious or frustrated. Someone who feels anxious and helpless to deal with the incident may cope with these feelings by reacting excessively or inappropriately.

# Inappropriate reactions

The person with dementia can be easily moved to tears and sometimes to bouts of uncontrollable crying for no apparent reason. Outbursts of laughter when the situation is sad or anger when the opposite response is called for are also examples of inappropriate reactions.

The person does not seem to be aware that the feeling being expressed is inappropriate and their odd reactions do not seem to have any effect on them and hardly, if ever, affect others. They may not be upset by gentle remarks, such as, 'Oh John, this is a sad story and you are laughing', but still will not recognise that the behaviour is inappropriate.

# Shallow reactions

Some dementing people are easily moved to tears, laughter or anger. There is no apparent depth of feeling and the expression of emotion is fleeting.

# Extreme reactions

The strength of the emotion being expressed is at times out of proportion to the situation. The person may have an aggressive outburst while being bathed or dressed, smash ornaments because they are 'in the wrong place', or pace frantically when expecting a visitor. On the other hand, some may react to a distressing situation by quietly refusing to eat or otherwise to cooperate.

### *Explosive outbursts*

Sudden outbursts of extreme emotion may take the form of:

◆ frantic pacing
◆ determined non-cooperation

◆ shouting, wailing or loud sobbing
◆ hysterics
◆ hitting, punching or biting
◆ throwing or smashing

These eruptive and sometimes dramatic outbursts are immediately noticed and usually receive urgent attention. If they are neglected, though, the outbursts will invariably worsen. Unless the situation or underlying cause of the anxiety is corrected, episodes of similar behaviour will happen more frequently and each incident will be more intense. This may lead to the person being sedated or physically restrained, the consequence of which may be significant complications.

### Quieter reactions

In some instances uncharacteristic quieter behaviours are also expressions of extreme emotions. They may take the form of:

◆ refusal to eat
◆ sleeplessness or nightmares
◆ sullenness or evasiveness
◆ listlessness
◆ negativism

Quieter emotional reactions such as these do not usually pose a problem, especially in residential care, and are often thought to be a characteristic of the dementing illness or part of the person's normal behaviour. They tend to be ignored and the person will often deteriorate physically. By the time the deterioration is noticed, the person may be ill, or living in a state of increasing isolation and intolerable anxiety.

# Try to find the reason

In some instances you may be able to identify the reason for the excessive emotional behaviour. You might find that it is a reaction to an upsetting incident or something that is causing frustration or fear. On the other hand, an underlying reason for the excessive reaction may remain hidden because the person does not know or is not able to tell you what happened to cause the anxiety.

If you observe closely, however, you may be able to identify the incident or person who triggers the extreme reaction, and take steps to prevent it happening again.

◆ Does it happen at the same time each day?
◆ Is it a reaction to:
—the same incident, person or situation?
—a change of environment?
—emotional stress: being lost or frightened?
—physical distress: pain, cold, heat, tiredness, hunger, a need to go to the toilet or insufficient exercise?
—delusions or hallucinations?

### *Cultural norms*

In many cultures it is normal to express feelings loudly and with vigour. Understand that this behaviour is not necessarily an overreaction to a situation, but the person may be acting in a way that is expected in his or her own culture.

## Specialist consultation

Where an extreme emotional reaction persists and where it is disruptive or dangerous to others, or harmful to the person themself, specialist psychological consultation should be sought.

---

### THE CATASTROPHIC REACTION

The nature of the catastrophic reaction is often misunderstood, mostly being used to describe sudden violent behaviour in people with dementia. This is not the full picture.

The theory of the catastrophic reaction was originally applied in biological science and has been adapted to a number of other disciplines, including aspects of human behaviour. Put simply it means that certain catastrophic events or stimuli that happen in a person's life will trigger a change in the way that a person acts.

In the treating of brain-damaged patients earlier this century it was found that when they were presented with a task or a memory that was too much for them, they would be overwhelmed, and anxiety and irritability flooded over them. They coped with these feelings by reacting with seemingly inappropriate and excessive emotions and behaviours. These took the form of restlessness, agitation, hyperactivity, anger, tremor, tears, determined refusal to cooperate or evasiveness (evasion can take the form of physical avoidance or emotional withdrawal). It was something like a panic attack that these people were experiencing.

Common catastrophic reactions of the person with dementia include frantic pacing, agitated and night wandering, aggression, crying, whimpering and hysterics, determined non-cooperation and emotional withdrawal. Of course these sorts of behaviours can happen for other reasons too, but it is the reason for the behaviour happening that separates a catastrophic reaction from other emotional or behavioural reactions.

It is important to understand the catastrophic reaction because we often unwittingly precipitate this reaction in people with dementia. Catastrophic reactions are less likely to happen if we avoid:

◆ presenting a task that is too difficult
◆ recalling distressing memories
◆ making sudden unnecessary changes
◆ applying physical restraint
◆ arguing or unduly insisting and reasoning

---

# Anecdotes of extreme emotional reactions

' Mild-mannered Mr Lim walks into the crowded sitting room, tearing furiously at fastenings and shedding his clothes as he goes.

Nobody told the nurse who dressed him this morning that, for some unknown reason, he has taken a violent dislike to the cardigan she insisted he wear.

---

In her broken English, Mrs Berger repeatedly tells staff: 'I worried … going to ask me leave … nowhere go.' If a member of staff accompanies her to her room, points to her name on the door and opens cupboards so that she can see and touch her clothes, she is content for a few hours.

On the other hand if she is ignored or told she is mistaken, she becomes agitated, noisy and demanding. She goes to her room, picks up the flexible shower in her en-suite bathroom and sprays around the room shouting, 'Not mine, not mine!'

---

Mr Jack's behaviour has worsened from disruptive to violent. He has no speech and bangs on walls with his fists, rattles doors and throws objects. Frequently he raises his hands to his mouth, grunting and glaring at those around him.

Sedation makes little difference and he is transferred to a hospital security ward. An observant nurse suspects he is in pain, and an abscessed tooth is diagnosed. After this is treated, much of Mr Jack's disruptive behaviour disappears.

---

Ten days after Mrs Payne comes to live at the hostel she still refuses to speak to staff or join in with residents. At night she resists going to bed and is often found wandering aimlessly in the early hours of the morning. Her family complains she ignores them when they visit, sometimes taking herself to bed, turning her back and pulling the covers over her head. She refuses to take the presents they bring.

Treated with understanding, and as she becomes accustomed to life in the hostel, her sullenness and uncooperative behaviour decrease.

# Antagonism between residents

A difficult reaction to deal with is aggression that results from provocation by, or antagonism between, residents.

In residential care these incidents will often occur at the busiest time of the day, when there is little or no supervision. If possible, roster on one member of staff to occupy residents with a quiet activity. Where antagonists are known, try to separate them as often as possible.

---

**Extreme emotional reactions are rarer in a calm environment with trained staff who are understanding and take a personal interest in the residents and promote a feeling of security.**

# CHAPTER FIVE

# Each person is unique

> 'In all the world there is no one else exactly like me. There are persons who have some parts like me, but no one adds up exactly like me.'*

## GETTING TO KNOW THE PERSON

No person with dementia is the same as another. Each is unique.

Understand the person as an individual as well as the illness. Get to know the 'who' as well as the 'what'.

The simplest way to begin to know the person is to:

—listen to what the person has to tell you

—talk to relatives

—obtain a functional assessment

—compile a personal profile

## Look for the person behind the illness

Knowing how a dementia illness affects the person helps you understand why someone behaves in certain ways. However, for

* Virginia Satir, *Self Esteem*, Celestial Arts, Berkeley, Ca.

professional care workers to provide the best possible quality of life for each individual we need to know 'who' the person is as well as what the illness is.

### Listen to the person

A good starting point to begin to know the person is to listen to what they have to tell you. You might be surprised how much you can learn about a person over time, by engaging them in conversation. Even if the person has limited ability to carry on a conversation they might well be able to indicate likes and dislikes or even things that interest them, in a non-verbal response to your suggestions.

### Talk to families

The home carer will be able to supply you with valuable information about the person's interests, what they respond positively to and what upsets or annoys them. Families have known the person for many years and their contribution in helping you to know the person as an individual is invaluable.

I have always found relatives agreeable to providing information about the person who is to be accommodated in a residential care facility. Generally families are pleased, even gratified, by the staff's interest and are reassured that every attempt is being made to understand their relative.

## The functional assessment

A functional assessment will indicate what the person is capable of doing, what they will do and where they need help. One of the priorities for the use of the functional assessment is to encourage the affected person to continue to do what they can do and make allowances for what they are no longer able to do.

An occupational therapist or gerontological nurse attached to an Aged Care Assessment team, hospital or memory disorders clinic, particularly if they know the person with dementia, is often the best person to do this assessment.

# The personal profile*

Completing the personal profile before the person moves to a hostel or nursing home gives staff information that will help with the new resident's adaptation to new surroundings and circumstances.

The personal profile will further help to individualise the person. The information gathered will give a picture of where the person grew up and lived, family, interests, likes and dislikes. It provides cues for conversation and prompting of memory. These are some of the areas to look at when building the personal profile:

◆ the person's interests
◆ what she or he likes to talk about
◆ the person's values
◆ what they like to do—gardening, farm work, housework, chatting, crosswords, listening to music, watching football, and so on

## *View videos and films*

Many families have films and videos of their relative at a younger age and viewing these will add another dimension to 'who' the person is.

> The staff of the nursing home accepted Louise as nothing more and nothing less than an Aboriginal lady with specific symptoms of dementia who needed their care. One day her daughter brought a video which showed Louise as a highly articulate lobbyist for Aboriginal women, moving with ease amongst a social gathering at Parliament House. They developed a special interest in Louise from then on and related to her in an entirely different manner.

By the time the care worker has gathered some of this information they will begin to understand the person as an individual. The person will no longer be only the woman or man who has dementia and who needs care. Instead they will be seen as a husband or a wife, a father or a mother, a soldier who served in the war, a grandmother who made tapestries for all of her grandchildren, a coach of the soccer team, a ballet dancer.

---

* See Appendix A.

*Important note to families and professional workers*

1  Do not include any information on general files that is confidential or likely to be misinterpreted.

2  Add current information from time to time.

3  Staff should explain to families how the information they give will be used, for example that all staff and volunteers will have access to it.

# SELF-IDENTITY

A person's identity is the 'self', the 'me' who is unique.

The way we perceive our 'self' influences the way we behave and how we fit into life around us.

As the dementia progresses the identity of the person disintegrates.

Parts of the identity or 'self' may persist well into the illness and be preserved by the affected person:

—playing out life-roles

—clinging to habits

—retaining a sense of humour

—confabulating

—presenting a social front

Sometimes the identity is distorted.

# The 'self'

We are all aware of having an identity, a 'self', a 'me', who and what we are and where we fit into the pattern of life around us. We have an image of ourselves and we act according to the way we perceive our self-image.

The 'who' and what we are is moulded by our life experiences and the roles we fulfil. Our self-esteem and the satisfaction we feel about ourselves is added to by other people's positive attitudes to us.

As dementia worsens, the affected person will become progressively confused about who they are; self-image becomes blurred and personality falls apart. Consequentially self-esteem diminishes and confidence is lost. Others will totally lose their identity and no longer be aware of who they are.

## Parts of identity may be retained

Some parts of the identity, however, may be preserved and the person may retain some sense of who they are well into the illness.

> Eighty-five years old, mother, grandmother, great-grandmother and ex-owner of a beauty shop, little Mrs Goode is confused. She cannot read or write now and becomes lost if she goes out alone.
>
> Yet she has a strong identity as the matriarch of four generations of a large and loving family, an image strengthened by their attitude towards her. They visit often and include her in family gatherings. She remembers some of the family gossip and enjoys recounting family doings to interested staff. Her self-esteem is high.

## Distorted identity

Because of confusion and memory loss, the person with dementia often has a distorted image of 'self', not being too sure of their identity or where they fit into the world. This distortion may happen occasionally or be incorporated in the ongoing personality.

You will often get the impression that the person struggles mentally to maintain their 'self' and by responding seriously to the way they see themself, especially when they appear to be struggling mentally, you will help them to maintain a self-image and enhance their integrity and dignity. On the other hand, if the person's concept of 'self' is ignored, mocked or sternly corrected, they tend to become more confused and are at risk of prematurely living in a vacuum.

> In the nursing home Mrs Spring, 79 years old, lives out her earlier identity as a young woman. She waits impatiently for her children to return from kindergarten, concerned that 'they must have missed the bus'. She 'sets' the table and cannot understand why her husband is late for dinner.

When she is reminded of where she is, that her husband visits her daily and her grown children have families of their own, she looks perplexed and becomes silent and withdrawn. But by sharing her concern and encouraging her to talk about her family, her agitation eases.

On occasions, Mr Adams reverts to a strong identity as a business executive. Believing the dementia hostel is a hotel, he asks the 'maid' to 'Please bring me a fresh towel' and orders room service. He asks that a phone be connected in his room so that he can make business calls. Polite and dignified, he resents being told or ordered to do things and corrects staff if they use his first name or call him 'mate'.

Staff respond to the identity he believes in, treat his requests seriously and politely explain that the rules of 'this hotel' do not allow private telephones.

## How identity is preserved

The person with dementia will preserve remnants of their identity and self-image by:

◆ playing out life-roles
◆ finding a new role
◆ clinging to habits
◆ retaining a sense of humour
◆ confabulating
◆ presenting a social front or veneer

# LIFE-ROLES AND HABITS

**Throughout our lives we play many roles: son, daughter, parent, student, employee, spouse.**

**Life-roles help to establish our identity.**

**The dementing person may retain one or more of their life-roles.**

**Some people create new roles for themselves.**

**Self-esteem is enhanced when the role the person presents is recognised.**

**Habits are automatic actions or practices that are part of everyone's day-to-day life.**

**People affected by dementia gain security from clinging to habits, although sometimes the habit is inappropriate or harmful and control is necessary.**

# Life-roles

At any one time we fulfil many roles: daughter, wife, mother, employee, neighbour, friend, business executive or secretary of the tennis club. Some roles are short-lived, some life-long. A person who is affected by dementia may still cling to one or more of their life-roles.

## *Roles confirm identity*

Roles give us a place in life and are part of our identity. They confirm a sense of being 'me'. Our life-roles can make us feel useful and important. Little Mrs Goode (in the anecdote on page 72) plays a life-role that still exists, and one that strengthens her sense of identity and enhances her self-esteem.*

> Every morning Mr E. dresses and sets off to catch the bus to the business he used to own. He becomes irate when his wife tries to convince him that his business has been sold long ago. She devises a scheme:
>
> She watches while he puts on a clean shirt, tie and suit and checks his briefcase and kisses him goodbye when he leaves. After giving him time to arrive at the bus stop, she drives past and then, feigning surprise to see him there, she offers to give him a lift to 'work'. She drives him around for a while, sometimes stopping off to have a cup of coffee, then she takes him home. His role is confirmed and the daily hassles cease.

*See previous section on self-identity.

In the anecdotes on page 73, Mrs Spring's role of young wife and mother and Mr Adams' role of business executive survive only in their minds. Their behaviour is inappropriate in the present circumstances but they feel important because staff treat them with dignity and respond to the roles as they present them.

> Miss P. plays out the role of her previous occupation of matron of a small private hospital. You can imagine the sorts of difficulties this creates for both staff and residents in the dementia hostel where she lives. Locks need to be installed on the treatment room and office doors to prevent her 'treating' other residents, answering phones and tampering with files. Explanations have to be given to the visitors who are 'interviewed' by Miss P.
>
> To stop her frequent visits to the staffroom and reproaching staff for being idle, the 'STAFF' sign is relocated to the door of her room.
>
> Several techniques that are familiar to her are devised for diverting her energies. Counting and stacking linen, and keeping daily 'records' of the furniture and appliances in the recreation room are tasks which she happily does over and over, occupying much of her waking hours and preserving her self-image.

## *Finding a new role*

It is not unusual for a person with dementia to find a new role for themselves. Be sensitive to signs of this happening and encourage the person who tries to establish a role for themself either at home or in a residential facility. Carrying out a special role gives a sense of achievement. You may even find that a person will develop a sense of ownership of a role and become upset if another person tries to take it over.

> After a few sessions Irene memorises the sequence of morning exercises and establishes herself in the role of prompter. Quick to remind the recreation worker when an exercise is missed, she glows when the group looks to her for guidance.
>
> ─────────
>
> Several times each day Tom takes Heather and Mavis for walks in the garden. He opens the door and takes one of them on each

arm. Leading them into the garden, he is careful to avoid overhanging branches and rough spots on the path. When he is praised for the role he has undertaken his broad smile indicates his pleasure.

———

We were making a video in the nursing home which the residents all seemed to enjoy.

But at three o'clock every afternoon Jean would confront the crew: 'I'm in charge here,' she would say, 'and I would like you to go now.' If we didn't pack up immediately, she would insist: 'These people have had enough of you, and you've had a fair go. Pack up and leave! Now!' Jean had temporarily assumed the role of supervisor and protector of the residents.

## *Creating a role*

With a little imagination you can create roles for people by using their interests, remaining skills and capacities. You will need to be prepared to remind and supervise them.

Animal-lovers Phyllis and friend John accept the staff's request to look after the dog. They spend happy hours brushing and walking the gentle Labrador. Supervision is needed, otherwise they would save their meals to feed to the dog.

———

Lily is the biscuit-server at morning and afternoon tea. Emma and Kate are table-setters and Marie wipes up. Frank is the vegetable-grower, gardening in his own special patch. John replaces the chairs after the exercise group.

———

Mrs Toller, who runs her small bookkeeping business from home, encourages her husband, Dennis, to fulfil the role of letter collector. He waits eagerly for the postman each day and brings in the letters and opens the envelopes. Several times during the day he checks the box for newspapers and pamphlets. His wife has to oversee his activity otherwise he will feed everything through her paper shredder.

# Habits

Habits are actions or practices that have become automatic through repetition. They are a familiar part of our day-to-day behaviour and are one of the aspects that go to make up our identity.

### *Clinging to habits*

By being able to indulge lifelong habits, the person with dementia feels comfortable and safe. How often have you observed the woman contentedly dusting furniture, wiping tables or sweeping the floor, or the man who watches football on television, even though he no longer understands the rules of the game?

> As a sales manager, Mr Grant frequently ate in expensive restaurants. At the day centre, having no money to 'pay' for his meal and leave a tip for the 'waitress' distresses him. He eats little. His wife supplies him with some coins, thus restoring his dignity—and his appetite.
>
> ────────
>
> Miss Perkins causes a commotion each evening when she refuses to shower. After consulting her sister, we restore her lifelong routine of showering in the morning and dressing 'ready for work'. The problem is solved.

### *Habits that are not appropriate*

It is not always possible or appropriate for someone to indulge their habits. Sometimes pursuing the habit can be harmful to a person who may not always appreciate the reason.

> Every time Sophie leaves her room in the hostel she dresses in an afternoon frock and best shoes, just as she did when she went out from her home. Her foot becomes infected, but despite the discomfort, she still refuses to leave her room if she is not wearing the shoes. On the occasions we succeed in persuading her to wear special soft shoes, she soon returns to her room to change.
>
> Finally we 'lose' the best shoes on top of her wardrobe until the foot heals. Sophie wears her slippers, complaining continually.

# HUMOUR, CONFABULATION AND SOCIAL FRONT

A sense of humour, confabulation and a social front add to and confirm the person's sense of self and feelings of importance.

A person affected by dementia may retain a characteristic sense of humour. Laugh with them.

Confabulating eases the person's anxiety by providing an explanation for what they do not understand or cannot remember.

A social front is also called 'social veneer' or 'social facade'.

A social front exists when the person retains conversational skills, good appearance and manners.

The social front may mislead the onlooker into believing that nothing is wrong with the person.

## A sense of humour

A sense of humour helps us to deal with the ups and downs of life. Because a person affected by dementia may tend to lack expression or have difficulty with words, we do not expect them to be humorous but some have a great capacity to see the funny side of things.

### Retaining characteristic humour

It is true that some people never develop a sense of humour. But where someone had a sense humour before the dementia, it will invariably continue to exist for a considerable time into the illness.

Some people with dementia have the capacity to perceive the subtlety of a funny situation or to make a witty remark, even though much of their intellectual functioning is diminished. Sometimes even the speed of the repartee will surprise the listener.

A sense of humour is a very personal attribute and varies from person to person. Even if whatever is amusing the person is not immediately understood, nevertheless respond to the 'joke'. Entering into the fun lightens the person's life, amuses others and gives a feeling of importance and of being appreciated. Laugh with people, not at them.

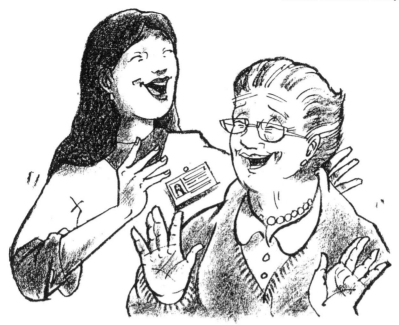

> Bill has a whimsical sense of humour. He can no longer walk, but he delights in telling the occupational therapist: 'My wife is bringing my dinner suit so I can take you dancing tonight.' They share the joke.
>
> ———
>
> In the film, *I Remember Love*, the wife, although aware of her dementia, hides objects and then forgets where she has put them. One day when she walks into the kitchen she comes upon her husband searching for a baking-dish. 'You too?' she queries. Then seeing a funny side, she bursts into laughter.
>
> ———
>
> Mary has a sense of the ridiculous. She loves to play the clown, trying on funny hats or mimicking staff.

## Confabulating*

Confabulating helps to confirm the person's identity by filling in memory gaps and providing explanations for what is not understood.

---

\* Read this section in conjunction with 'Delusions, hallucinations and confabulation' in Chapter 3.

It added to Bill's sense of importance when his doctor believed that he was an officer in the Army Reserve.

───────

'I am only here for a few days for a rest, you know. I really must go home,' the neat 55-year-old Elma informs the new volunteer. She talks about her career as a professional musician. She confides that she is feeling better after the rest 'here', but now needs to go home to practise her violin to perform in a concert next month. Elma's story is so believable that the volunteer approaches the manager to have her discharged.

In fact, Elma used to be a children's music teacher but has not taught or played her violin for many years. Inventing her 'story' helps her maintain her sense of being 'someone', as well as explaining to herself why she is in this strange place.

### *Acting out the confabulation*

Sometimes confabulating is accompanied by the person's acting out of a role.

Mr P. tells everyone at the day centre he is there to fix the plumbing. Even though staff know he has not worked as a plumber for many years, they know that he is well satisfied that they treat his story as real.

On her first day the volunteer gives him a spanner so that he can put in a tap washer. She returns to find him gazing helplessly at bits of tap as water gushes out, flooding the kitchen.

## A social front

The person who presents a social front or a social veneer retains conversational skills, pleasant manners and often a neat appearance.

Visitors to the dementia unit are delighted when Vera Henry greets them: 'I am pleased to see you.' She may offer to show them over the unit or ask them if they would like a cup of tea. She talks about the weather or tells them about her family. Strangers often question whether she should be in residential care at all because it appears that there is nothing wrong with her.

––––––––

Four people sit together chatting animatedly. Heads nod and hands wave to emphasise a point, just like any social gathering. But if you listen, you will find the conversation makes little sense. They are even speaking different languages!

### *A social front is deceptive*

'The new care worker asks why Mr Peel is in the special unit. 'I don't believe there's anything wrong with him. He's so polite. He pulls up a chair and opens the door for me and I just had a long chat with him about football.'

This is a common reaction when this sort of veneer exists. The person's demeanour and social skills mask the characteristics of the illness and give the appearance of normality. When you pursue conversations, though, they seldom make sense. Nevertheless this social veneer is valuable in that it helps to maintain social relationships and so confirms the person's identity and adds to their enjoyment and self-esteem.

## WAYS TO CONFIRM IDENTITY

You can help keep the person's identity 'alive'.

Use the person's name. Talk about their life interests.

Personal possessions, full-length mirrors, neat appearance and a little flattery help confirm a person's identity.

A pleasant and interested attitude on your part adds to feelings of being valued as a person.

Encourage independence and praise achievements.

# Confirm identity

You may not be able to slow down the progression of dementia but you can help to keep the person's identity 'alive' while it still exists.

## *Use names*

Always start a dialogue with someone by using their name. Repetition of someone's name confirms that person's identity both to themselves and others.

## *Talk about life-roles and events*

Spend time talking to the person about 'who' they are, for example: mother, husband, career woman, football coach or friend. A person who is still able to converse will often initiate a discussion about themselves or their experiences. Encourage them to talk about themself. Also take every opportunity to mention past and new life-roles that give them pleasure: 'Mrs Frazer, your daughter's had a new baby? You're a grandmother again! Congratulations!' or 'Mr Jackson, you did a great job helping me empty the waste paper baskets this morning'.

Even the smallest recognition of a personal nature will confirm identity and add to the person's self-esteem.

## *Familiar activities*

Activities that are familiar to the person are more likely to stimulate recollections of 'who' the person is and their life experiences and so reinforce their identity. Gather information about the person's interests and previous activities and provide opportunities for them to pursue as many of these as possible.

## *Personal possessions*

Photographs, ornaments, personal toilet articles, cosmetics, clothes, an old bank book, cheque book or coins in a purse or pocket all confirm identity. A much-loved jacket, handbag, shopping basket, the briefcase carried to work for years or a bunch of old keys are part of the owner's body image. Remove them and you disturb the person's perception of 'me'.

' Mrs Quell brought into the hostel a cloth bag in which she kept a conglomeration of articles: sewing cottons, a change purse, an old wallet and cheque book, chocolate wrappers, two books, and so on. So closely she guarded it; placing it firmly in her lap when she sat and carrying it around by its two enormous plastic handles everywhere she went.

Disaster struck when she was transferred to the dementia unit of the retirement village where she lived and the bag was mislaid. It was as though Mrs Quell had lost an extension of herself. She paced frantically, looking for it everywhere, rummaging through the possessions of other residents, throwing cushions from chairs and upturning mats and generally being disruptive. When she tired of searching, she would sit alone and talk to no one.

When the bag turned up Mrs Quell was overjoyed and regained her friendly and talkative nature. That bag was an important part of Mrs Quell's identity. '

## *Money*

Allowing the person to have money is always a somewhat contentious issue. Money will often 'go missing' in residential care facilities and relatives rightly complain that they cannot afford to provide money when there is no supervision. Staff equally rightly feel that they should not be expected to accept responsibility for the safety of money.

Possessing money has great significance for some people. You only have to observe the expression on the face of the woman who checks her change purse occasionally or the contented look of the man who jingles the few coins in his pocket. One man convinced his wife that the lottery tickets he gave her were dollar notes and she was happily able to 'tip' the staff of the dementia unit for their 'service'. On the other hand, in one dementia unit when some of the residents were provided with plastic play-money 'to spend', they weighed it in the palms of their hands and deciding that it was too light, rejected it.

Where providing a person with money has a positive outcome some arrangement could be negotiated between staff and family to supply a few cents for the person's use.

## *Personal appearance*

Attention to clothes, a weekly visit to the hairdresser or barber, an occasional manicure and a little flattery enhance a person's self-image and contribute to a good feeling about themselves. Hairdressing and nail manicuring are usually carried out in the unit. Some units employ hairdressers; others have hairdressers visit regularly, while other residents are taken to the salon either by a family member or staff. Nails are usually attended to by volunteers or included in a residents' activity program.

There are some nursing homes or hostels who encourage residents to select their own clothes and have one of the stores bring a selection to the facility. Staff may take a few chosen ones shopping for this purpose.

Shopping expeditions can be fraught with difficulty. In his numerous talks, Gordon Sweetman, a well-loved member of the NSW Alzheimer's Association, would tell this story about his wife, Iris. It went something like this:

> We were on our usual shopping expedition to the David Jones store and Iris went into the fitting room to try on a couple of dresses. It was sale time and the department was full. To my horror and to the horror of customers and the young sales assistant, Iris appeared at the entrance of the fitting rooms clad only in her bra and panties. I grabbed a dress from the closest rack and covered her. It all turned out quite well though, when I explained to the salesgirl in a good loud voice that Iris had Alzheimer's disease and didn't always know what she was doing. Did I stop taking her to the store? Well no, she enjoyed those outings and after that I would get one of the sales assistants to go with her to try on the dresses.

## *Mirrors*

Full-length, impact-resistant mirrors also help to maintain a person's interest in their appearance and reinforce body image. However, there is some debate about the provision of mirrors in facilities where people with dementia are accommodated. The opponents of access to mirrors are concerned that a person who hallucinates may see a frightening image and strike at it, smashing the mirror and injuring themselves. It does seem a pity though that the number of people who might gain some satisfaction and benefit from viewing their images should be deprived on account of one or two at risk. It would seem to be more effective to prevent the person at such a risk from having access to the mirror and to make certain that all mirrors are impact resistant.

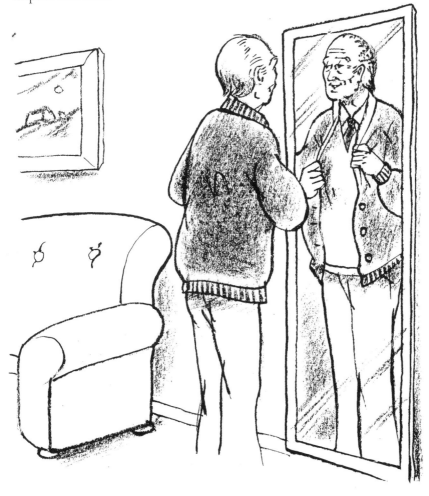

# Your attitude is important

Your positive attitude can help to preserve the person's identity and heighten self-esteem by making him or her feel worthwhile and needed.

Our beliefs and values and attitudes are moulded from birth by our family, our religion, our culture and the generation we belong to. This means that there are wide differences in values and attitudes particularly in a multi-cultural society such as Australia. In a nursing home or a hostel you may find several different sets of values amongst staff, and it is usually the attitude of the individual staff member that determines the way the resident is treated.

Understanding and acceptance of the values and attitudes of each resident by all staff is of paramount importance for their wellbeing.

### Be courteous and interested

Treat the person with dignity and respect; as an adult, not as a child. Be courteous. Be interested. Value what the person is telling you. Listen and respond; do not brush it aside or ignore it.

### Give choices

Multiple choices can be confusing and frustrating, but people with dementia are usually capable of making simple choices. Offering a choice gives the person a sense of control over their life.

◆ 'Would you like me to call you Ruth or Mrs Pearce?'
◆ 'Mrs Jackson, which dress would you like to wear?' (showing only two dresses)
◆ 'Cyril, do you want to watch TV now?'

### Allow feelings to be expressed

Recognise a person's feelings, do not ignore them. We often try to make someone 'feel better' by soothing a troubled person: 'Don't worry about it, it's not important'; 'I'm sure your daughter didn't mean to be nasty'. But these sorts of comments may make the person feel that you do not understand or, worse still, that you do not care about them as a person.

*Empathise* if someone is sad, irritated, angry or depressed: 'I can see that what John did made you mad'; 'It's pretty upsetting when someone says something nasty to you'. People with dementia have a range of emotional responses and even if sometimes they are inappropriate they need opportunities to express these feelings.

## Respect privacy

Everyone needs a patch of their own. Respect personal space and possessions: 'Is it OK for me to turn your radio down?' Always knock and ask, 'May I come in?' The person may not answer, but will understand your attitude.

## Explain what you are doing

Explain what you are doing or what you are about to do with the same consideration you would show to others in your own home or to your friends. Explaining has the added bonus of including the person in what is going on in the world around them.

- ◆ 'John, I'm putting your clean clothes in your drawer.'
- ◆ 'That's my brother at the door. He's taking me home.'
- ◆ 'I'm going to play a tape. I like band music.'
- ◆ 'Doris, walk with me across the room.'

## Encourage independence

Encourage independence wherever it is possible. Appreciate, however, that there are times when the person feels insecure or frightened and needs to be dependent on you until their anxiety has passed.

## Praise

Praise even small achievements, neat personal appearance, good behaviour and eating habits. Praise adds to self-esteem and may lead to a repetition of the behaviour praised. Praise must be sincere.

CHAPTER SIX

# The problem-solving approach to handling behaviour

I have chosen to use the term 'problem behaviour' rather than the politically correct term 'challenging behaviour' currently in use, for reasons set out in the Introduction.

The way the person with dementia acts can be roughly divided into:
—symptomatic behaviour
—pre-morbid, or previous, behaviour
—environmentally-provoked behaviour

Behaviour only becomes a problem if it is harmful or overly distressing to the person with dementia or to others.

In most cases the person cannot help or control strange behaviour and disruptive actions. They are caused by the dementia illness.

The intensity of the strange behaviour and disruptive actions diminishes as the disease progresses into the final stages.

Medication often has no effect on problem behaviour.

Problem behaviour is often the consequence of a wider problem situation.

Handling problem behaviour requires the development of special skills.

Be calm, confident and consistent.

A problem-solving approach is likely to provide long-term solutions to problem situations and provide clues for prevention.

The person must not be punished under any circumstances.

When we talk about behaviour we simply mean the way that everyone acts or conducts themselves in everyday life. In this chapter and in Chapter 7, we deal with a number of situations and behaviours associated with people with dementia that can often be frustrating, stressful and difficult to handle. Some of these behaviours are just strange and perplexing, others are disruptive and frightening, while some can be harmful to the person themself and to other people. While some people can be demanding and disruptive, most are merely vague and confused and, in the main, gentle.

It is important to differentiate between the way we perceive behaviour that is volatile and is a problem, such as aggression, which must be contained or prevented, and that which is just strange and sometimes difficult to cope with, such as repetitiveness, which in the main we have to accept.

If we are to develop skill in handling behaviour that causes problems both in the home and in residential care, we need to have some understanding of the behaviour of people with dementia. To do this, I have attempted to tease out the threads of dementia behaviour into three separate but often overlapping categories:

1  symptomatic
2  pre-morbid or previous
3  environmentally-provoked

## Symptomatic behaviour

Many of the behaviours that people with dementia exhibit need to be considered entirely as symptoms of the illness. Or, to put it another way, 'normal' for the illness. These behaviours will vary from person to person, and will occur regardless of whether or not we intervene, although in instances where there is a problem, steps have to be taken to handle it. By the time a very severe stage of dementia is reached, all behaviour will be symptomatic.

Examples of symptomatic behaviour are: muddled actions and conversations, aimless wandering, becoming lost, some instances of inertia (listlessness), repetitiveness, brain time-clock sleeplessness and loss of social control and so on (see Chapter 5). The man who does not recognise his wife or his home does not act this way on purpose. It is a symptom of the illness. He cannot remember them. Aggressive reactions can be symptomatic when associated with certain types of dementia illnesses.

Marginally associated with symptomatic behaviour are the person's physical condition and emotional state, delusions, hallucinations and depression or symptoms of mental illness.

## Pre-morbid or previous behaviour

It is not unusual for a person to retain some of his or her characteristic way of acting for some time into the illness. Bits of behaviour will be exactly the same as they were before the person was affected. For example, the gardener may still do a good job of weeding the vegetable patch and the woman may still read her paper each morning. The person who used to pursue solitary interests may strongly resist being included in group activities in residential or day respite care. Someone who regularly bathed at night may be uncooperative if asked to shower in the morning.

Previous behaviour may become distorted or exaggerated, for example the habitually tidy person may develop an organic orderliness, constantly tidying up or laying all sorts of objects in neat rows or in strange and unusual arrangements. People who previously reacted to certain situations with irritation may become cantankerous or aggressive. The woman who reads the paper may go through the motions without understanding what it is that she is reading.

Even though this type of behaviour is distorted it will still bear traces of the way the person behaved before. Of course not all previous behaviour is desirable and it can on occasions cause difficult situations, such as the erstwhile dependent person who now clings and follows staff and residents at every opportunity. Or the man who was an active walker, who now has no sense of location, but takes a hammer to the lock on his front door so that he can escape.

Where it does not create problems and while traces of this sort of behaviour remain, provide opportunities for the person and encourage them to maintain their characteristic behaviour.

# Environmentally-provoked behaviour

Environmentally-provoked behaviour is much more complex than the previous two and much more 'problem behaviour' lies under this umbrella than is generally recognised. However, because of its nature, this behaviour is often easier than the other two to modify and prevent.

Where a problem is provoked by environmental factors, as well as being profoundly affected by dementia, the reason for the behaviour, the core of the problem, lies elsewhere. It may be the consequence of provocation by another person, or even because of our actions and the way we react to the person. It may be associated with an emotional upset with a relative or with the tone and atmosphere of conversations or activity going on at the time. For example, the death of a resident or a staff conflict can affect the mood and behaviour of everyone in a residential facility.

Rather than concentrating on the behaviour alone, we need to take a much broader and more detailed overview in order to find a solution. In the discussion later in this chapter on the problem-solving approach, I suggest ways in which this can be done.

# What is problem behaviour?

Behaviour that is strange or irrational is not necessarily a problem although it is often seen as being so. As a general rule, *problem behaviour* is behaviour which causes the person with dementia great unhappiness or which accelerates their deterioration, or behaviour that is harmful to themselves or others.

Each person will exhibit or react with his own particular range of behaviours and these may be frequently repeated. In many instances it may be the way the person has always dealt with stress; it may be uncharacteristic; or it may be due to a catastrophic reaction.

Problem behaviour frequently occurs towards evening. There have been many reasons suggested for this. It has been observed that difficulties occur at this, the busiest time of the day, perhaps as a reaction to the quickened pace in the unit. Tiredness may be another contributing factor: tiredness of the person with dementia, weariness of the carer. Whatever the reasons, the behaviour puts added pressure on the home carer or the residential care worker. If the person is severely scolded or restrained, this may have no other effect than to make them more distressed. Or if medication is administered to control the behaviour, it often meets with little success.

## Use of drugs to control behaviour

Drugs are commonly used to modify behaviour that is seen to be a problem or which staff are not able, or do not have time, to handle.

'Medication mostly has no effect on problem behaviour associated with dementia, particularly Alzheimer's disease. In fact, medication may have severe side effects and cause more problems than the behaviour itself.'*

There is now a groundswell of opinion that controlling behaviour with drugs designed for the treatment of mental illness is not desirable. Tremor, unsteady walking, leaning, falling, injury, drowsiness, blurred vision, dry mouth, loss of appetite, incontinence, and increased confusion and memory loss are some of the possible side effects of medication. Sometimes the medication itself can cause or increase disruptive behaviour.

Medication *does* benefit behaviour associated with some forms of depression, symptoms of psychiatric illness and sleeplessness, and dosages should be monitored regularly.

## Physical restraint to control behaviour

Tying people into chairs, sitting them in bean bags so that standing is difficult, locking them into chairs with lap trays are methods used in some residential facilities to control behaviour that is difficult to contain. Together with drug control, physical restraint is undesirable and can have severe psychological, emotional and often physical consequences for the person who is restrained.

---

* Dr Helen Creasey, Staff Specialist Geriatrician, Sydney University/Concord Hospital, New South Wales, private correspondence.

## GUIDELINES FOR RESPONDING TO PROBLEM BEHAVIOUR*

Sometimes appropriate responses will modify undesirable behaviour. You might find the following suggestions useful:

◆ Be confident. Understanding the reason for the behaviour will help you cope.

◆ Be calm. Speak quietly and do not retaliate.

◆ Be firm. Let the person know the behaviour is not acceptable.

◆ Approve and praise acceptable behaviour.

◆ Be consistent.

◆ People who are in residential care accommodation are usually more content and are less likely to be disruptive where:

—staff understand the effects of dementia illness

—the resident is treated as an individual

—the atmosphere is caring and the routine flexible

—surrounding and activities are familiar

—staff have good communication skills and the capacity to step into the strange, confused world of the person with dementia

# No one way of dealing with problem behaviour

It is patently clear to most people who have lived or worked with people with dementia that there is no one effective way of dealing with all dementia behaviour, or even a single way of responding to any one behaviour. Neither is there is a single solution: one situation can be surprisingly simple to deal with while another can be extremely complex and the resolution difficult. Various techniques and 'therapies' have had some degree of success: the spaced retrieval technique in particular has proved to be effective in some instances. Discouraging unacceptable behaviour while consistently approving acceptable behaviour and diverting attention may bring about some improvement. A warm, caring atmosphere with a minimum of negative stimuli goes a long way towards preventing behaviour that is difficult to cope with.

* See Chapter 7 for suggestions for dealing with common problem behaviours.

Some of these techniques are often the only reasonable option for dealing with certain types of difficult behaviours, particularly that of a symptomatic nature. However, in most instances they provide only temporary relief at best and are not likely to have a lasting effect. Most of the behaviours will recur and we are left with the task of having to deal with the problem over and over again. For many behaviours that are problematic, particularly those of an environmentally-provoked type, a more permanent solution is possible by applying the problem-solving approach.

# THE PROBLEM-SOLVING APPROACH

Why does the problem behaviour happen? How should I respond? How do I prevent it? How do I find the best possible solution? These are the questions to ask when using the problem-solving approach.

When we focus solely on a person's behaviour, what we are trying to fix can simply be a symptom of a larger problem situation. The behaviour doesn't get any better, or, if modified, soon recurs. Instead of targeting a behaviour alone, the problem-solving approach deals with the whole situation. It looks at a network of factors: the circumstances that contribute to the problem, the interactions of everyone involved and the consequences of these dynamics.

The problem-solving approach can be likened to a photographic shoot where the camera operator uses a wide-angle lens to include the background, the scenery and the people as well as the main subject of the picture. Similarly the problem-solving approach broadens the focus to take in the whole scenario and all the players. As well as assessing the dynamics of the whole situation, this method avoids the pitfall of laying blame on resident, staff or family which can happen when we look at undesirable or 'challenging' behaviour in isolation. The problem-solving approach:

1   moves the emphasis away from the person involved and focuses on the reason for the behaviour occurring or the core of the problem;

2   concentrates on a problem *situation* rather than a problem behaviour;

3 does not use words such as *managing, controlling* or *challenging*;
4 uses terms such as *circumstances, problem situation, strategies* and *responses*.

## Planning the problem-solving approach

There are three steps in planning the problem-solving approach:

1 Defining the problem.
2 Assessing the person in the situation.
3 Planning a strategy to solve the problem.

### Step 1: Defining the problem

◆ *What is the problem?* Is it the behaviour of the person with dementia? Family dissatisfaction? Staff attitude?
◆ *Whose problem is it?* Is it a problem for everyone: staff and family, the person with dementia, or just one person? Sometimes we label a certain behaviour as a problem because it does not conform to our beliefs and attitudes about values and the proper way to act, or because we find it uncomfortable or difficult to handle. But these are *our* problems and not necessarily problems for others, or for the person with the dementia. *We* may be the solution to the problem.
◆ *What is the desirable outcome?* Make a group decision as to the very best outcome for the problem. Take, for example, the problem of someone who refuses to shower. The desirable outcome would be that the person cooperates with showering.
◆ *What is the* tolerable *outcome?* Of course we would all like to achieve the perfect outcome, but this is not always possible. So consider also an outcome with which everyone concerned will be reasonably satisfied. In the case of the person reluctant to shower, a shower three times a week and a sponge bath on four nights might be a tolerable solution.

---

**At the end of Step 1, we now have an overview of the problem and a clear objective to work towards.**

---

## *Step 2: Assessing the person in the situation*

This next step is to make an assessment of the person, together with all the factors that may contribute to the problem situation. We are now looking for the core of the problem and the circumstances that trigger the behaviour. Ask: *'What is happening to make this a problem?'*

*Assess the person* Problem behaviour is often directly associated with physical or psychiatric factors. Do not overlook these.

◆ Is the person:
—unwell, in pain, troubled by dentures?
—overtired, overstimulated, bored, anxious?
—embarrassed, ignored, misunderstood, feeling patronised?
—delusional, hallucinatory?
or reacting to:
—an unpleasant incident or association or change?
—a disturbing memory, or a personality conflict?
◆ Is the behaviour the only way the person can communicate with you?

Where possible, ask the person with dementia their opinion of the problem.

*Assess the background* Sometimes there is some experience or other factor in a person's background that is clashing with their present circumstances. Look at:

◆ race, culture, upbringing, socioeconomic status
◆ morals, religion and other values
◆ pre-morbid personality and home behaviour (consult the family)

*Assess the situation* Look at every factor possible in the situation. Sometimes it is the most unlikely thing that is the reason for the behaviour.

◆ When and where does the problem happen?
◆ Does the behaviour always happen in the same place? In similar

surroundings? Is there something in the surroundings? Does it always happen with the same person or in similar circumstances?

◆ Who are the other people involved—staff, visitors, family, a friend, another resident?

---

**At the end of Step 2 we have a pattern of the problem. We have identified the behaviour that everyone finds a problem; we have decided on a tolerable outcome; and we have assessed all the other contributing factors. We have discovered the core of the problem and the trigger for the behaviour. We can now plan a strategy to respond to the problem.**

---

## Step 3: Planning a strategy

In planning the way in which we are going to respond to the problem, we need to take into account all the resources that are available to us.

◆ *Resident*: How much does the resident comprehend? Can they contribute to the solution? Can using the person's likes and dislikes, skills, habits, and so on contribute to the solution? How much can other residents contribute?

◆ *Family*: Family, particularly the home carer, is the most significant and helpful resource. Family members have lived with the person with dementia for a lifetime, and have looked after them during the earlier stages of the illness. They may have dealt with this problem before. How much can they contribute with information or intervention?

◆ *Staff*: Is there one member of staff who has already solved the problem? One who has the most influence with the resident? One who comes from the same cultural background?

◆ *Outside agency*: Is there an outside agency or organisation that can assist? Cultural factors may be the key. Outside leisure or religious activities may be part of the solution.

---

**By now you have enough information to design a successful strategy to solve the problem.**

---

# Problem solving in action

An example:

> It seems as though Mrs Prim will never run out of excuses for not taking a shower: 'Yes dear, I will have a shower, but not just now'; 'I'm just waiting for my daughter, I don't want to miss her'; 'Yes, I will have a shower in the morning/tonight/after lunch'; 'Well, dear, I just want to watch "This Day Tonight" on TV'. Staff cajoled, persuaded, bribed, diverted, threatened, forced. Nothing worked. But they would often find her half-clothed trying to wash herself from the hand basin. Staff agreed that the tolerable outcome would be for Mrs Prim to shower without fuss four days a week and that they would work towards this.
>
> An assessment of the problem situation revealed that Mrs Prim had always been a very independent person. She was particular about her appearance and belongings. She was in excellent physical health and appeared to enjoy living at the hostel. Information from her daughter, previously the family carer, included that Mrs Prim was in the habit of using a special set of towels and matching face washer and only one brand of soap; she didn't like to have her hair washed under the shower, and some years before she had fallen while showering and broken her wrist. Since then she was fearful of another fall. There had been no problems with showering while she was at home.
>
> There was another problem. For no apparent reason she was particularly difficult with one personal care assistant and refused to even talk to her. Her daughter was able to supply the reason.
>
> This personal care assistant whom Mrs Prim appeared to dislike bore a marked physical resemblance to a woman with whom her husband had had a brief affair, many years before. Staff took the following steps to solve the problem.
>
> ◆ The daughter agreed to shower her mother while a member of staff observed.
> ◆ The same routine was followed in the future:
>   —using a towel, face washer and special brand of soap brought from home;

—encouraging Mrs Prim to gather them together to take them to the shower herself;

—providing a chair for her to sit on in the shower recess and a non-slip mat to stand on;

—encouraging her to wash and dry herself, only helping where necessary;

—washing her hair in the hand basin, using her own shampoo; arranging regular visits to the hairdresser.

After following this routine a few times, Mrs Prim agreeably showered every day. As for the personal care assistant, when she realised that there was nothing personal in Mrs Prim's dislike for her, her own attitude changed. She set about to slowly impress her own identity on Mrs Prim.

Two techniques she used are to constantly identify herself to Mrs Prim and to find time to tell her anecdotes about her own life.

Here are two more brief examples:*

After weekly mass in the nursing home, Mr Bass is overcome with extreme hunger. Nothing less than a cooked meal will satisfy him, even though he has eaten a hearty breakfast less than an hour before. Staff reason with him and point out that he can never manage to do more than pick at the second meal anyway. All to no avail. He becomes agitated and abusive. (This was identified as the problem behaviour.)

On applying the problem-solving approach, staff are able to identify the core of the problem. It is the priest who provides the clues. Mr Bass only remembers the time when it was not permitted by the Church to eat after midnight on the day before mass, and his mind is still experiencing the intense hunger he had felt then. The problem is solved by putting half of Mr Bass's breakfast aside so that he can eat it after the mass.

———————

Mr and Mrs Bright were depressed. Antidepressants had little

* See Appendix A for documentation of this problem.

effect. Both suffering from early/moderate Alzheimer's disease, they were housed in a secure dementia unit. They withdrew from the other residents and only reluctantly joined in some of the group activities, although it was known that they had previously enjoyed a socially active life.

After applying the problem-solving approach, the solution was to find a volunteer from the local Returned Servicemen's League (RSL) Club, who accompanied them to the club every week, so that they could pursue activities in an atmosphere that had been a major part of their lives for many years. There was a remarkable change in their mood and attitude.

## The advantages of the problem-solving approach

As well as promoting a happier environment for both the person with dementia and staff, and at times resulting in a more satisfied family, this method leads to a decrease in the incidence of problem behaviour. A most important benefit is that it provides clues to prevent the behaviour from recurring.

Other advantages of the problem-solving approach are that it:

◆ focuses on the person in a problem situation, rather than on the behaviour;
◆ offers another option for dealing with difficult situations;
◆ provides an added skill for professional workers;
◆ avoids negative terms such as *managing, challenging* and *controlling*;
◆ talks about:
   —problems and problem situations
   —assessing the situation or looking at the circumstances
   —solving and finding a solution
   —responding to the person
◆ removes the concept of 'blame' from the person with dementia, the family and the worker;
◆ is the most effective way to deal with situations that involve interpersonal relationships;
◆ provides clues to prevent the behaviour from recurring.

# CHAPTER SEVEN

# Frequently occurring problem behaviours

There are times when a behaviour that is causing a problem requires an immediate response. In this chapter we look at the nature of some behaviours that occur frequently when people are affected by dementia, and examine how some of these should be handled:

◆ anger and aggression
◆ attention seeking (looking for love and care)
◆ repetitiveness
◆ non-cooperation and negative reactions
◆ losing, hiding, accusing, rummaging, pilfering and giving away
◆ evening agitation and sleeplessness
◆ eating
◆ sexual behaviour
◆ loss and grief

## ANGER AND AGGRESSION

**Angry and aggressive behaviour may be a symptom of dementia.**

**Anger and aggression can occur for other reasons. The person may become annoyed or angry if she or he feels:**

**—not understood**

**—rejected**

**—frustrated**

**—provoked**

**—patronised**

**Aggressive behaviour is more likely to occur at a time when the person is:**
—overtired
—overstimulated
—under-exercised
—uncomfortable
—ill

**Try to prevent aggressive behaviour. Aggression can be minimised if you:**
—are calm
—do not shout or retaliate or restrain the person
—avoid situations you cannot handle
—assess your attitude

**Deal with anger, then divert the person's attention.**

# Anger

We all become annoyed or angry sometimes. People with dementia are no exception.

Mrs Benson rushes from her room, her face flushed and her pencil-slim body taut. Her usually clear speech is almost incoherent: 'That ... that woman ... ' She points to the woman who frequently raids her wardrobe and who today is wearing her shoes and cardigan.

Mrs Benson's anger melts when we return her clothes and accompany her while she puts them in her drawer. If we brush her aside or do not intervene she will do physical battle with the offender to retrieve the garments.

# Aggression

If anger is not handled and modified, it may develop into aggressive behaviour: shouting, throwing or destroying things or attacking people. Once you are familiar with the person, however, it is easier to identify the sorts of situations that will precipitate the aggressive behaviour and attempt to prevent it occurring.

## When does aggressive behaviour occur?

Aggressive behaviour is more likely to occur when the person is over-tired, overstimulated, under-exercised, uncomfortable, ill or in pain.

## What triggers aggressive behaviour?

Aggressive behaviour is triggered by:

◆ unresolved anger;
◆ misunderstanding;
◆ rejection;
◆ provocation;
◆ personality conflicts;
◆ being patronised or belittled.

## Who might become aggressive?

The person most likely to engage in aggressive behaviour is one who:

◆ is frustrated by having insufficient speech to be understood;
◆ cannot comprehend what you are asking;
◆ is suspicious and hits out to protect from imaginary threat of harm;
◆ has a strong irrational dislike for another person;
◆ has always reacted to stress with aggressive behaviour.

## The person who is not understood

Is the person becoming agitated because they are not able to make you understand? If what they are trying to tell you does not make sense, do not give up. Be patient. Sit with them, keep intermittent eye contact and assure them you are trying to understand. Look for clues: an occasional word, a gesture or a facial expression. Your understanding of the situation and knowledge of the person may provide a hint. Your patience and reassurance will mostly prevent escalation of the anger.

## Show the person who is not understanding

If the person is becoming angry because they cannot comprehend what it is you are asking, show them. For example, if you are asking them to move to another place, stand near the chair and beckon, patting the seat of the chair, 'Jack, would you please sit in this chair?' If Jack still does not understand, gently take his arm and propel him towards the chair: 'That's good!'

Practise asking yourself, 'How can I show him?' You will be surprised at how creative you are.

# Hitting out

> Chairbound Mr Murphy, ex-boxer, complains that diminutive Miss Walker is going to hurt him. He threatens her with his walking stick when she wanders into his room. Once, in terror, he hits her and knocks her to the ground. Reasoning with him is useless. He persists in his belief that he must protect himself from 'this evil woman'.
>
> It is impossible to control Miss Walker's wandering, so she is moved to a room on a busy corridor where staff are passing frequently and can monitor her movements. Now that Mr Murphy sees Miss Walker only at mealtimes, when staff are present 'to protect me', he feels secure and is much calmer.

Racial tensions are often transported with the person when they leave their country of birth. Combativeness between residents can often be on account of these tensions.

> Karl seems to take a violent dislike to Uri from the day they first attend day care. Karl provokes Uri by shouting abuse in German. Uri shouts back in Russian and punches Karl. Maybe Uri is mistaking Karl for someone else; maybe he reminds him of some disliked person from his past. It could be a hangover from a deep-seated cultural conflict.
>
> The day centre arranges for them to attend on alternate days and neither shows any signs of aggression.

Irrational dislikes seldom improve. They seldom respond to reason. If they are allowed to go unchecked, they invariably explode in physical combat. In the nursing home or dementia hostel, separation of the antagonists may be the only safeguard, allowing them to come together on the fewest possible occasions.

## Suggestions for responding to aggression

Sometimes aggressive behaviour cannot be avoided or prevented. In most instances, however, it can be handled in such a way that it does not endanger others. Try these suggestions:

◆ Avoid the situation. Until you become confident, aggressive behaviour can be scary. If you feel insecure when you are faced with an enraged person, slowly move away, first making sure others are not in danger. Call someone nearby for assistance, if possible.

◆ Be calm. Take a deep breath to relax your body. Slowly move in front of the person, speaking gently. Your tone of voice is important, but the words you use are of no consequence. Repeat the person's name quietly or say, for example:
—'Dulcie, it's all right, it's all right. Don't be scared/upset.'
—'No, no. NO. NO.'
—'Anne, please stop. You are frightening me/poor Mrs Jones.'

◆ Engage the person's eyes and keep talking quietly. Do not make sudden movements, stretch out your hand or touch the person. This may be interpreted as an attack.

◆ When the anger begins to dissipate (this may take several minutes) tentatively touch the forearm or, with your palm upwards, invite the person to hold your hand. Walk with them or wheel them if chairbound.

◆ The person will settle but do not leave until you are sure the likelihood of another explosion is over.

### *Do not provoke violence*

Shouting, ordering and retaliating are likely to provoke violence, to you or someone nearby. Grasping the person or otherwise restraining them puts you in danger of attack. Goaded by rage, the person will invariably have more strength than you.

### Reasoning

Because aggressive behaviour is irrational, it seldom responds to reason. This does not mean that you should not tell the aggressive person the behaviour is unacceptable: 'Mr Peck, you upset/frighten me when you are angry.'

He may get the message, and you will certainly feel better.

### Is it you?

If you are a worker in a residential unit and you attract more than the usual amount of aggression from residents, you may need to assess your attitude. The solution may be simple. Or you may not really enjoy working with people with dementia and would be happier transferring to another section.

### Sedation

In most cases, to control aggression fully it is necessary to administer sufficient medication to keep the person in a sleep-like state. This is undesirable, for it deprives the person of any life at all. Medicating after the outburst has passed accomplishes nothing. There are other ways to handle aggression, as set out above.

## Anecdotes of aggressive behaviour

Mr Peck is a fearful sight when he is infuriated. He shouts unintelligibly, his face contorting in a horrible grimace. The recreation worker, determined not to reveal her apprehension, avoids him. One day, unable to escape, she is confronted by Mr Peck, arm raised to hit her. She tells the story:

> I was rooted to the spot, then suddenly I became aware of a look of indescribable sadness in his eyes and sensed in him a terrible feeling of desolation. I was drawn to him and the expression on my face must have communicated my empathy. I remember saying something soothing and reaching for the hand by his side. His body relaxed, the threatening arm slowly lowered and he smiled at me. He must have remembered because he wasn't ever aggressive with me again.

‘
### *Rejection leads to aggression*

It is shift-change time. Everything is going wrong. At her desk the supervisor, already late, hurries to write up files before handing over. For the fifth time in as many minutes, she looks up as Mrs Black complains about lost spectacles:

'Oh, go away, Mrs Black. Can't you see I'm busy? I told you before, I haven't got time now to worry about your glasses.'

Mrs Black takes off her shoe and hammers, heel down, on the desk, breaking a vase.

Mr Newman receives a similar answer when he asks about his medication. Stomping away from the desk, he shoves a man who has accidentally bumped him. The man staggers and falls.
’

Both incidents might have been avoided had the supervisor replied, 'I know you're worried about your glasses/medication. If you wait a few minutes I'll get someone to help you.'

### *Turn a minus into a plus*

A potentially dangerous situation handled sensitively may be turned to advantage. A minus can be turned into a plus.

‘
Everyone is at breakfast except Mr Granowski. He is energetically gathering chairs and stacking them on one side of the recreation room. Mr Granowski used to be a furniture storeman and all his activity now centres around the unit's furniture. Nobody knows what makes him so agitated. It could be frustration at no longer being able to communicate, even in his native Polish.

Now, grasping his arm and pulling him away from the chairs, the new cleaner shouts at him to stop. Mr Granowski takes a swing at her. Momentarily the cleaner grapples with him. Mr Granowski picks up a chair and aims it at the window.

Enter a nurse. She speaks softly until he becomes less active, then she takes him by the hand and strokes his arm: 'Thank you for stacking the chairs. Now let's put some around for the others when they come.' She works with him.

As well as averting a violent incident, the nurse gives Mr Granowski a sense of usefulness and importance. Remembering her, he rises from his chair each time she enters a room and invites her to sit. This is undoubtedly his way of recognising her understanding.

**,**

---

**Deal with the anger first, then divert the person's attention.**

---

# ATTENTION SEEKING—LOOKING FOR LOVE AND CARE

**People who engage in attention-seeking behaviour such as clinging and following and crying out are looking for love and care.**

**Rename it 'looking-for-love-and-care' behaviour.**

**This behaviour may be a reaction to discomfort, loneliness, fear or the inability to communicate needs.**

**To reduce grasping, clinging and following:**

**—provide company**

**—divert the person to a group activity**

**—encourage the person to take part in a physical activity such as walking**

**To decrease the incidence of crying out, make them comfortable and provide company.**

We often have negative feelings about people who are demanding or who engage in attention-seeking behaviour. The offender is often ignored or scolded because we believe that 'giving in' will make them more persistent.

In a residential facility other people may only be able to cope with the demanding behaviour by avoiding social contact with the person, criticising, and even sometimes retaliating with physical abuse. Unsatisfied and rejected, the person's self-esteem diminishes and behaviour worsens.

## Looking for love and care

The first step towards responding to attention-seeking behaviour is to rename it 'looking-for-love-and-care' behaviour. You might find that your attitude will soften you and that a cheerful word and a hug is sufficient to satisfy the person.

## Crying out

Frequently, demanding behaviour is a reaction to discomfort, loneliness, helplessness or an inability to make oneself understood.

'Hostel residents are exasperated by Mrs Cryer's continuous calling, 'Hullo, hullo.' They either shun her or call her names. On occasions, a distracted resident hits or shakes her. She responds neither to coaxing nor to rebuke. When she is seated at an isolated table during meals and away from the others in the sitting room, her shouts become louder. She seems to gain perverse satisfaction from the reaction to her increasing use of lewd words.

Mrs Cryer has Parkinson's disease. She is able to walk slowly but has difficulty rising from a chair. After sitting for long periods, her limbs become stiff and painful, and she has too little speech to communicate her need to move.

When she is helped to stand and stretch every half-hour and is taken for frequent short walks she is more comfortable. A pleasant remark from everyone who walks past means that she no longer feels overlooked. Apart from the occasional lapse, Mrs Cryer's demanding outbursts cease. '

The person who cries out or shouts continually is usually one who is confined to a chair, although often the reason is not as obvious as the circumstances in Mrs Cryer's case. All that we can say is that if the crying out is ignored it will persist. On the other hand by attending to the person, making sure that they are not cramped, in pain, wet or dirty and providing them with company, the behaviour will lessen.

# Grasping, clinging and following

Grasping, clinging and following is another irritating and difficult behaviour to handle. It often persists throughout the person's waking hours and alienates residents, as well as trying the patience of staff and the home carer. Where the behaviour is mild, attention can be diverted by encouraging the person to join an activity group, or providing any other form of occupation.

Because grasping, clinging and following is often a trait of the agitated walker, they can seldom remain in an activity or interest group for long. If they are safe and not made more anxious, leaving them to walk outside in a secure area may keep them occupied for some time.

If you sit or walk with the person, the behaviour will lessen. However, as this sort of behaviour is often continuous, most of us do not have this much time to spend with one person. It is rarely possible to prevent clinging and following because there seem to be no specific reasons for the behaviour.

> As the volunteer passes by, Mr Smith grasps her arm, digging in his nails. He pulls himself from the chair and with a steel grip shuffles alongside the volunteer, babbling unintelligibly. Everyone avoids him and some of the frailer residents even fear him. The only respite for staff is when he is eating or sleeping.
>
> Staff of the dementia unit plan to deal with Mr Smith's behaviour by paying him more attention. Before he is able to grab them, they take his hand and walk along with him. Anyone with a minute to spare sits with him and he is encouraged to walk with others in the garden.
>
> It is difficult to assess how effective this is in allaying Mr Smith's anxiety. The moment he is left alone, he reverts to the demanding, clinging and following behaviour. However, staff gain a sense of satisfaction because they are coping, and fewer occurrences of the behaviour mean there is less tension for everyone in the unit.

# Volunteers

Hard-pressed staff of residential facilities seldom have the time to devote the amount of attention needed to the person who is continually demanding and volunteer visitors are reluctant to undertake this task. One nursing home designed a project appealing for volunteers especially to spend some time with three women who were continually crying out. They offered some training to help them understand these women and offered continuing support from a trained staff member.

No volunteer was expected to spend more than two hours with the women, which meant that several people were necessary if the program was to be effective. The volunteers decided that one volunteer at a time would accompany the three women as a group.

They read, played music, talked, wheeled them out or just sat with them. It is uncertain how much the women understood of what was being said or read to them, nevertheless they sat quietly. Not only were the women quiet when the volunteers were with them but staff reported that they seemed more content and overall the noisy behaviour had noticeably decreased.

# REPETITIVENESS

When memory is severely impaired, what happens from moment to moment may not be remembered. Also, the part of the brain which signals when to stop activity may be damaged.

The dementing person may engage in the same activity, tell the same story or ask the same question over and over again.

Provide articles the person can fold, stack and sort. Keep cloths and brooms handy for wiping, dusting and sweeping.

Listen to the story as though it is the first time you have heard it.

Deal with repeated questions seriously and politely.

Modify any factor in the environment that may reduce anxious repetitiveness.

Paradox: A person who does not remember may still be able to reason.

# Repetitive behaviour

When memory is severely impaired someone may not recall what happens or what they have said from moment to moment. Also, once having started an activity the brain may no longer have the capacity to tell a person when to stop so that they may repeatedly engage in the same activity, retell the same story or ask a question again and again and again.

## *Repeating an activity*

Folding, stacking, sorting, wiping and dusting are some of the activities most often repeated, although you will also notice that some people will repeatedly engage in other activities or repetitive actions. Hand movements and ritualistic walking patterns are also sometimes repeated.

For those who like to fold, helping to fold towels, face-washers and clean laundry seems to be a satisfying occupation. Plastic plates and magazines are suitable for stacking and plastic cutlery for sorting. Also provide boxes of colourful material remnants or containers with an assortment of articles.

In some residential facilities, domestic-type activities are not encouraged, for the simple reason that many staff do not approve of people doing 'housework' when they grow old. You will often hear a care worker say, 'I don't want to be doing housework when I'm old, I've had enough of that all my life. And I don't think you should expect other people to do it.'

What is being missed here is that some people have always taken a pride in their houses, and it is a spontaneous action of the 'houseworker' who gets satisfaction from the activity. If you look closely in a scene in the video 'Dementia with Dignity', you will see a woman resident in the background, busily cleaning with a carpet sweeper, an activity she will do for long periods. This woman also delights in helping to hang out the washing and other domestic chores.

## *Repeating a story*

'Nurse,' Miss Simmons sparkles at the occupational therapist, 'did I show you what I won at bingo?'

'And Nurse,' calls her friend Betty, 'did you know my daughter came to see me this morning?'

'So you're both happy, eh?' the OT responds for the umpteenth time. She knows nothing will be achieved by reminding them they have repeated their good news for the last two days to everyone willing to listen.

## *Repeating a question*

Sometimes irritating and difficult to deal with is anxious and repetitive questioning.

'Gerald, that's the tenth time in five minutes you've asked me about your medication,' the young personal care assistant sighs, rolling her eyes to the ceiling. Glances from those around indicate they know exactly how she feels. Gerald is satisfied when they tell him he has already taken his pill, yet he reappears immediately at the nurses' station with the same query.

Even though Gerald cannot remember what happened a moment ago, he does remember the names and dosages of his medication, reading the names from an old prescription. Noting that he can also read his watch, the psychiatric nurse plans to teach him to monitor the times for his medication.

On two pieces of white cardboard she draws large clock-faces, using the same numerals as those on his watch. The hands point to dosage times. The cardboard clocks are attached to the wall behind his bed. Staff take every opportunity to repeat the 'lessons' and each time Gerald asks about his medication, someone takes him to his room to read his clocks.

Soon Gerald is observed comparing his watch with his cardboard clocks. He tells staff, 'At eight o'clock I have my pills.' He is proud of his achievement. He does not always get it right and from time to time anxiety surfaces and repetitiveness returns.

## *'If he can reason why can't he remember?'*

A paradox is the person who on the one hand is mindlessly repetitive, but on the other appears able to reason.

James is transferred to the dementia unit, while his wife Clare remains in the hostel in the same grounds. James has a poor memory. He approaches one person after the other: 'Excuse me, I wonder if you can help me? I'm worried about my wife. I'm afraid she is ill.'

He is not convinced when told Clare left a few minutes ago. He reasons, 'If my wife isn't ill, she would be having lunch with me. I think you're just telling me she's all right to stop me worrying ... You say my wife lives here and you don't know the number of her room? I don't believe you. You're treating me like a child!' A moment later he says to the same person, 'Excuse me, I wonder if you could help me?'

Some of his anxiety is relieved when Clare changes her visits to late morning and stays for lunch.

Do not be discouraged if you cannot limit repetitive behaviour. Like most strange behaviour, it will pass.

# NON-COOPERATION AND NEGATIVE REACTIONS

**There is usually a reason for uncooperative behaviour.**

**Make sure what you are asking is understood.**

**Is it necessary for the person to do what you are asking?**

**Uncooperative and negative behaviour can be minimised by:**

**—leaving and trying again later**

**—diverting attention**

**—quietly insisting rather than asking**

**There are several techniques to coax the person to take therapeutic medication.**

**A person may become uncooperative or negative for a time after moving to a nursing home or hostel.**

**You will encourage trust and cooperation if you are reasonable and patient.**

# Uncooperative behaviour

In most instances when a person is not cooperating with what is being asked of them, there is a reason. Check the following:

◆ Can you be heard and seen?
◆ Is what you are asking misunderstood, too difficult or unfamiliar?
◆ Is the person suspicious of what you are asking?
◆ Has something upset them?
◆ Are they having a catastrophic reaction?

Reluctance or refusal to cooperate is usually due to one or more of these reasons. If what you ask is reasonable and you are patient, the person will soon trust you and is more likely to cooperate.

> The man who in his native country bathed infrequently refuses to shower in the hostel. Instead of insisting, we persuade him to have a daily wash assisted by a male care worker. Gradually he cooperates and showers willingly most days.

## *Says 'yes' but does not do it*

When someone agrees to do something and then does not do it, they are not usually being uncooperative. They may not understand what you are asking them to do. Try showing what it is you expect.

Similarly, those who answer 'No, no' to everything you say are probably not being negative. They may not understand.

## *Does it have to be done now?*

Very few tasks have to be done immediately; with some it does not matter if they are not done at all. When someone is uncooperative, resisting or argumentative, reasoning is not likely to have any effect. Leave; then come back and try later.

## *Divert attention*

You can usually overcome the person's reluctance to cooperate by talking to them or diverting attention in some other way, while you involve them in the task at hand. If you anticipate someone is going to refuse to cooperate, walk with them for a while or engage them in a pleasant activity, and resistance will invariably disappear.

### Insist rather than ask

It is always preferable to ask for cooperation, but if the task is necessary you may need to insist. Even in instances of determined non-cooperation, the person may readily concur if you quietly and firmly insist rather than ask. Take the person gently by the arm and at the same time explain what you are going to do: 'Jack, I am going to help you have a shower now.'

## Therapeutic medication must be taken

Life-saving and therapeutic medication must be taken. Reluctance to cooperate in this case may indicate suspicion of a change in medication, for example liquid replacing a pill, or a tablet replacing one of a different colour and shape. Wherever possible, the medication prescribed should be in a familiar form.

If this is not possible, a trusted member of staff will usually be successful in persuading the person to take necessary medication. Alternatively, time dosages to coincide with visits from a close family member. The medication will soon become familiar and you will be able to revert to a normal routine.

Mixing medication with a sweet or jam works with some people. If someone is bothered by the unfamiliarity of trolley dispensing, try giving the medication in the privacy of their room. Try to avoid administering medication between mouthfuls of food at mealtimes.

Determined non-cooperation may be due to a catastrophic reaction.

## A negative personality

Everyone in the hostel tries unsuccessfully to cajole Mr Frewen to participate in activities, just as his children have been in the habit of doing.

'Mr Frewen, are you coming with us on the bus trip today?'
'No.'

'We'd love you to come.'

'No.'

'Mr Frewen, would you like a piece of cake with your tea?'

'No.'

'It's your favourite cake.'

'No.'

Persevering usually strengthens Mr Frewen's negative reaction but if he is left to his own devices, he joins the bus queue or helps himself to the piece of cake.

**,**

## Is it a reaction?

Determined non-cooperation and negativism are often reactions to a person's moving into a nursing home or hostel. Or they may be upset about something that is happening, or that they *think* is happening, in their lives.

With your understanding and assistance it will pass.

## LOSING, HIDING, ACCUSING, RUMMAGING, PILFERING AND GIVING AWAY

A person with dementia may simply have no memory of where they put a lost article.

When possessions are lost, suspicion and accusations of theft are commonplace.

Rummaging, pilfering and hoarding are not done on purpose.

Someone who generously gives away possessions has no control over the behaviour.

Management suggestions include the following:

—limit the amount of clothing and possessions

—mark clothing, possessions, dentures, spectacles and hearing aids

—provide diversions

—seek the co-operation of relatives

Where several people live together in a residential facility, keeping track of clothing and personal possessions can be an awesome task.

## Losing, hiding and accusing

Residents are continually losing possessions. They hide them in out-of-the-way places for 'safety': money in socks, dentures in the fruit bowl, in other people's rooms. Or they put them down and simply forget where they are. Sometimes the articles are permanently lost, being flushed down the toilet or put in with the garbage.

The suspicious person hides possessions in order to protect them from theft. They will not remember later and will accuse someone, often a disliked person, of stealing the article. No amount of reasoning will convince such a person that the article has simply been mislaid or that they have never had it in the first place.

Sometimes a resident insists that a member of staff or another resident has stolen their property. If relatives are also convinced of the staff member's 'guilt', as well as the time spent in searching for the 'lost' article, the staff member may be put in the unpleasant circumstance of having to justify their innocence to the supervisor or manager of the facility. If another resident is targeted as the 'thief', staff will invariably be called on to intervene in a combatant situation between the accuser and the accused.

## Rummaging and pilfering

This scene will be familiar to many:

> A middle-aged woman makes her way into a room, moving purposefully towards the bed in the corner. She tidies the top of the bedside table and turns her attention towards the cupboard, searching and raking through clothes and toilet articles in the drawers. She puts on a jumper and pops a framed photograph into her pocket.
>
> Before she finishes folding and replacing the clothes the chairbound occupant of the room is shouting, wielding his stick

and pushing her away. Confused and frightened, the rummager stands helpless.

The woman's behaviour is automatic: she is going through the motions of a task she carried out many times in her role of wife and mother. She does not mean to steal the jumper and the photograph but she can no longer distinguish between 'mine' and 'yours'.

# Hoarding

Hoarders may have a cupboard full of shoes, a collection of spectacles or a conglomeration of articles belonging to themselves and others. Scraps of paper may be saved or piles of magazines stacked in drawers or on shelves. An odour may lead you to an accumulation of food and flowers, sometimes hidden among underwear or shoes.

Where a person is known to hoard, regular inspections of likely places are advisable.

# Giving away

Giving away possessions is as difficult to control as pilfering.

'I can't afford to keep replacing my mother's underwear. She doesn't have a petticoat to her name and the knickers I put in her drawer yesterday have gone. Someone even stole the jacket I bought her last week,' complains Mrs Stamp.

Mrs Stamp's mother has 'adopted' the lady in the room next door and insists she wear her outer clothing and shoes (her mother is size 22 and next door is size 10!). She shuttles between the rooms with armfuls of underclothes, regardless of how often staff return them.

It is almost impossible to stop Mrs Stamp's mother giving away her clothes. Sometimes she can be persuaded, but forcing her to stop precipitates an aggressive reaction.

# What to do about it

There is not a great deal that can be done to prevent this sort of behaviour, but it can be modified.

## Limit quantity of clothing and possessions

◆ The possibility of loss increases the more clothing and possessions a person has.

◆ Store out-of-season garments with a relative or friend.

◆ The minimum amount of clothing the person can manage on depends on laundry arrangements. Sufficient outer clothing for seven days is usually adequate if there are no problems with incontinence or spilling food.

◆ Discourage the keeping of jewellery and valuables other than a wedding ring.

◆ If the wedding ring is loose, place it on a larger finger.

◆ Two pairs of spectacles are an advantage. Keep one pair in safe storage to be used while you search for the lost pair.

## Limit access

◆ Lock one side of the wardrobe containing at least half the clothing. Explain to residents what you are doing and involve them in decisions where possible.

◆ Firmly attach framed pictures and photographs to walls.

◆ Ornaments and personal belongings, placed where they can be touched, add to the person's identity and contentment. In extreme circumstances, however, you will need to balance the benefit against the risk of pilfering and breakage.

## Mark everything

◆ Mark everything! Sew on name-tapes or indelibly mark underwear, pantyhose, both socks, each shoe and slipper, brushes, combs, electric razors, outerwear, raincoats, cardigans, and so on.

◆ Attach an adhesive name label on each arm and outside bridge of spectacles and mark dentures and hearing aids with denture marker.

◆ Mark ornaments with waterproof pen. The owner's name should be marked on both the picture and the frame. This enables identification should they be pulled apart.

### *Provide diversions*

◆ Ransacking other people's belongings decreased significantly when one nursing home set aside an unused space for rummagers. A few racks of garments, a cupboard, a chest of drawers and a bedside table to hold clothes and soft items provide facilities for rummaging at will.

◆ Boxes containing shoes, clothing and material remnants, placed in living and recreation rooms, keep rummagers occupied.

### *Seek cooperation from relatives*

◆ Advise the responsible relative or friend of the rules regarding clothes and possessions. A printed sheet of suggestions to which they can refer is helpful.

◆ Explain the difficulties in monitoring clothing and possessions and preventing loss. Relatives may not be aware that this is a far greater problem in a unit than at home.

◆ Where incontinence or spilling causes the use of more clothing than the laundry system can cope with, provide access to a washing machine and drier. A relative or volunteer is usually happy to help out by putting through a load. This is preferable to storing an excessive amount of clothing.

◆ Ask families to sort through their relative's clothing regularly. Provide a receptacle for possessions that do not belong so that they can be re-sorted. Large plastic garbage bins are ideal.

# EVENING AGITATION AND SLEEPLESSNESS

**Agitated behaviour may increase in the late afternoon or evening.**

**If the behaviour is not contained, the person may have difficulty settling to sleep.**

**Difficulty in going to sleep may also be due to:**
—being in bed too early
—overstimulation
—overtiredness
—dozing and insufficient exercise
—fear
—pain

Damage to the brain sometimes causes the sleep pattern to reverse: the person sleeps during the day and is awake at night.

Noise, sickness, cramps, nightmares, delusions, hallucinations and wet clothing will interrupt sleep.

Avoid wet clothing by taking the person to the toilet before the bladder voids.

# Evening agitation

Towards the end of the day anxiety and confusion tend to increase. Pacing and wandering may intensify and the person may become irritable, noisy or more repetitive and persistent. In a unit, spasmodic arguments may break out; 'going-homers' pack bags ready to leave. Tiredness, vague associations with home and onset of darkness are said to contribute to evening agitation. However there are other factors that should be taken into account.

In a nursing home or hostel, evening agitation coincides with a busy time of day: change of shift, and evening bathing and meal preparation. If there are fewer evening staff the restless person will not have the same attention they enjoyed during the day. In the home, the carer is usually exhausted and often does not have the energy to devote to the demands of the person with dementia.

> In a nursing home where a recreation worker is rostered on late-afternoon shift, evening restlessness has all but disappeared. Quiet, supervised walks or other low-key activities keep residents occupied—and there. There is very little agitation.

Where restlessness in the evening is not contained, a person may carry the agitation over to sleep time and will often wander and disturb others.

# Inability to go to sleep

## *In bed too early*

Elderly people tend to get by on eight hours' sleep or less at home, often retiring at ten o'clock or later.

Moving from home to nursing home or hostel usually means a change of sleeping pattern. Often put to bed when it is still light, the person tosses and turns, repeatedly calls or gets out of bed and wanders. Medication induces sleep, but when the effects of the medication wear off the person will waken.

> In a special-purpose hostel one of the two evening nurses allows those who wish to stay up later to do so. She encourages a range of low-key activities: most stay on in the dining room with her, listening to music, chatting and looking at magazines. A small group watches television in a bedroom while the walkers roam at will. At nine o'clock they come together for supper, after which many drift off to bed.
>
> The need for medication decreases, wandering and other disturbances lessen and fewer changes of wet clothing during the night are required.

## *Overstimulation*

However, if the activity is too stimulating it can be counterproductive. A relaxed atmosphere should be encouraged. Avoid physical activity such as dancing, lively singing, bickering between residents or any activity that may produce excitement or nervous tension.

## *Overtiredness*

It has been suggested that if people are kept continually active during the day they will be so tired by nightfall they will sleep soundly. The tension created by keeping people 'on the go' all day, with excessive walking and other forms of exercise, tends to carry over into the night. Exhausted, the person is unable to relax sufficiently to sleep. It is preferable to keep to normal patterns of walking and activity.

## Day rest

For some, restlessness in the evening may decrease if they are encouraged to rest for up to an hour after the midday meal. However, continual dozing so that people do most of their sleeping during the day should be discouraged. When someone is allowed to catnap continually during the day it is unlikely that they will drop off to sleep easily at night.

Boredom and sedation are two of the most common causes of day sleeping. Regular exercise, and sufficient activity and interest to prevent boredom and enhance physical and emotional wellbeing will be of more help in promoting sleep than sedation.

Someone who is chairbound should not be isolated or left in front of television for long periods. In addition to routine walks, include this person in group walks, outings, activities and exercise sessions.

## Fear and insecurity

If the person is frightened or otherwise feels insecure, sleep may be impeded. Maybe an unpleasant incident during the day has upset them. Are they frightened of someone coming into the room? Cot-sides can be terrifying to someone who is not accustomed to them and does not understand why they are being used.

Moving from home to a nursing home heightens confusion and feelings of insecurity. Feeling lost and frightened, a person is reluctant to go to bed. They may get up and want to follow you around, disturbing others by calling out or trying to find a way out.

You may not be able to modify the underlying cause of the fear but you can reassure the person and stay with them until they are relaxed. A warm drink, a chat, a stroll and soft music, if it does not disturb others, will sometimes induce sleep. There is the person who because of anxiety or other reasons may have difficulty in sleeping in the seclusion of their own bed and be reluctant to go to bed. One effective way of dealing with this is to take him or her out of the room, settle them in a comfortable recliner-type chair, with television or radio on low volume. Mostly they will drop off to sleep in a very short time.

Introducing furniture from home will overcome many sleeping problems. Sometimes a person will sleep more soundly in the bed that they are used to; if they wake during the night and see familiar furniture and objects around them, this will sometimes alleviate feelings of insecurity. A night-light reduces anxiety.

### Interrupted sleep

Sleep can be interrupted by noise, sickness, cramps, nightmares, delusions, hallucinations and wet clothing. Calm the person's fears if they wake distressed. Persuade them to return to a warm, dry bed with a reminder that it is night-time. Stay until they settle.

### Wet clothing

It is sensible to limit the occurrence of interrupted sleep caused by the discomfort of wet clothing:

◆ Ensure that the person goes to the toilet shortly before the usual time of falling asleep.
◆ Over a period (possibly a week or two), determine the times the bladder usually voids.
◆ Wake the person ten minutes before the usual voiding time and take them to the toilet. The person will soon be asleep again and you will be saved the effort of changing wet sheets.

There seem to be two schools of thought about changing the sleeping person who is wet. One believes that it is preferable to allow the person to sleep on without disturbance. The other is of the opinion that the person should not be allowed to sleep in wet sheets and should be woken and changed.

## When night becomes day

This type of sleeplessness at night is a symptom of a dementia illness. Damage to the part of the brain that controls the person's automatic time clock (body clock) may cause the sleep pattern to reverse. Taking themselves off to bed after breakfast or during the day, these people will sleep most of the day and wake refreshed and ready for a night's activity. You can point out the clock, sun, moon and stars to convince them of the time, to no avail. You will not change the pattern.

### Staying up

In a unit where night staff are available, problems can be avoided by going along with this phase. The person is usually content to be with you, chatting or looking at magazines. Often they will tire about dawn or may even go to bed in the earlier hours.

You may need to supervise in case they wander or disturb others. Reverse sleepers often want to telephone family and friends in the small hours of the morning, engage in normal daytime activity or even dress ready for an outing. Provide a night meal: sandwiches, fruit and a glass of milk or a cup of tea.

### Advancing sleep

You could try to gradually advance the time for sleeping. Keep the person up an hour longer than the time they want to go to bed during the day, then push bedtime forward one hour each day. Eventually the person will reach a normal bed-hour.

## Sleeping problems at home

In the person's own home, sleeping problems can be difficult to handle. The carer who does not want to turn their life around snatches sleep where possible. Or, woken by the dementing spouse or anxiety about their safety, will sleep fitfully and become exhausted from lack of sleep. A relative or friend or a night respite worker in the home on a regular basis will provide the carer with much-needed rest.

Where the carer is still sleeping in the same bed as the spouse, consideration should be given to encouraging the carer to move out of the marital bed. Even a couple of nights a week of each week will provide some much needed rest.

---

**Ensure restful sleep. Provide a quiet atmosphere, exercise and activity.
Avoid boredom, overstimulation and overtiredness.**

# EATING

Meals should be served in a pleasant, relaxed and unhurried atmosphere.

Give a choice of food; you may have to help the person choose.

Encourage independent eating; provide aids where necessary.

It is possible to manage eating problems resulting from:

—reaction to changed eating patterns and unfamiliar food

—poor appetite

—unsatisfied hunger

—disruptive behaviour

Provide a separate area for people who are disruptive or primitive eaters.

It is not a good idea for dementing people to eat alone.

Outdoor meals are fun!

## Mealtime

Mealtime is a time for socialising. Serve meals in a pleasant, relaxed and unhurried atmosphere. Some home-like units encourage the residents who are able to collect meals from and return plates to the kitchen.

Tables, set with colourful tablecloths with only a little overhang, should seat no more than four. Clear plastic covers are easily cleaned and protect the cloths where there are likely to be spillages. Where table mats are used, some suggest that the colour should contrast strongly with that of the china so that it can be more easily distinguished. Medium-sized cutlery is more easily handled than large spoons and knives.

Provide paper serviettes for those who can manage them. For women who are likely to spill food, pretty aprons or smocks are preferable. These are no more trouble to launder than bibs which can be demeaning. For men, a serviette or towelling piece tucked into the collar, and if necessary one on the knee, usually suffices.

*Offer a choice*

Most people can indicate food preferences and a choice of meals should be offered. You may need to help some people choose.

*Outdoor meals*

Morning and afternoon tea, sandwich meals and barbecues are all enjoyable outside in good weather.

# Eating habits are hard to change

Before coming to live in a nursing home hardly anyone is used to eating daily in a dining room with twenty or more people. Meal routines may also be different: the evening meal at five o'clock instead of the usual seven o'clock; the main meal at midday instead of evening.

It takes time, attention and encouragement for the resident to adjust to the change. Some people settle more quickly if a relative or volunteer sits with them at mealtimes for the first few days.

## *Food tastes are acquired over many years*

Residents will often reject unfamiliar or bulk-prepared food. Do not insist on someone eating food that may be unappetising or foreign to them.

◆ Would a sandwich meal be preferred to the main meal?
◆ Will they eat the sweets or fruit?
◆ Does their religion have dietary sanctions?

People from other cultures may have great difficulty in adjusting to nursing-home food. In smaller units it may be possible occasionally to prepare a familiar meal. This does not mean opening a tin of spaghetti for the Italian person!

Where rejection of food is a serious problem, arrangements can sometimes be made with a relative to prepare tempting snacks or meals that can be frozen and used as required. Even a familiar sauce served with the meal stimulates the appetite.

Some facilities encourage a family member who wishes to do so to visit the unit, sometimes daily, to bring a familiar meal and, where necessary, to help with the feeding of their relative.

# Poor appetite

If the appetite is poor or the person refuses to eat, check that they are not ill or in pain.

◆ Is the problem a toothache?
◆ Are dentures ill-fitting, or lost?
◆ Is reluctance to eat due to medication or catastrophic reaction or depression?

# Encourage independence

Encourage independent eating for as long as possible. Be patient with the slow eater. Do not hurry him or her needlessly. This might result in someone swallowing unchewed food, choking or refusing to eat.

Very often a person is capable of eating independently but has lost the capacity to begin the actions for eating. You can encourage them by beginning the movements to eat: putting the spoon or fork in their hand may be sufficient to trigger the movement. If not, assist by guiding a spoonful of food to the mouth. If the person is able to eat independently, this is usually effective in beginning the activity. You may have to do this each mealtime.

## *Aids for eating*

Occupational therapists, or organisations such as Independent Living Centres, will be able to advise on aids to assist with eating. Some of the most common aids in use are suction cups to hold plates firmly, rimmed plates, purpose-designed cutlery, and double-handled cups and straws to assist independence with drinking. Contact occupational therapy departments through the local hospital or the Aged Care Assessment Team in your area.

# Feeding

If feeding is necessary, make mealtime as pleasant as possible. Sit beside the person, do not stand over them; and chat to them while feeding. Use a medium-sized fork or spoon. Do not overfill the utensil. Do not shovel: wait for the food to be swallowed before feeding the next mouthful.

Food should never be puréed or mashed unless the person cannot chew or has difficulty in swallowing or there is a medical reason. Encourage a choice—ask 'Do you want carrot now?', and hold up the fork spearing a piece of carrot.

> Nobody knows how much Ella understands. She has no speech. Usually disinterested in the world, she comes alive at mealtimes. Ella has definite food likes and dislikes. Mashing or puréeing her food results in unmistakable disapproval; jaws are clamped and she shakes her head vigorously until she receives a normal meal. She then signals her approval by nodding her head at each spoonful. Her pleasure at being understood and having her wishes considered is unmistakable.

# Always hungry!

Some people are always hungry. As well as their own meals, they will finish what others leave uneaten. After stuffing as much as possible into their mouths at morning and afternoon tea they will raid rooms looking for fruit and chocolate—or anything else that is edible.

Others will be hungry because they refuse to eat or have left the table without eating enough to satisfy the appetite. These people need to be more closely supervised at mealtime. On the other hand, it is common for someone to eat a satisfying meal and immediately forget they have eaten. But if you offer this person a biscuit or sandwich, they will seldom eat more than a bite. They will, however, be reassured that you treated the complaint seriously.

If there is a metabolic disorder, such as diabetes, restriction of some foods or quantity eaten is essential. Some over-eaters may become so obese as to cause health or management problems.

Because they are usually clever in obtaining forbidden food, persuading even strangers to bring them snacks, supervision is difficult but essential.

In some instances voracious eating seems to be associated with the brain damage; weight does not increase and the person remains healthy.

## Agitated behaviour

Anxieties often surface around mealtimes. Agitation is likely to increase when there is a delay between the residents being seated and meals being served.

> After five minutes, Mr Jessel jumps up and paces in the corridor. At the same table, Miss Becket shouts to the nurse. Mr King searches for his wife, who is probably at home, and refuses to eat 'until I find her'.
>
> This situation improves when they are moved closer to the kitchen and the meal is served as soon as possible after they are seated. Mr King's wife is asked to change her visiting time to mornings and arrangements are made for her to eat with him.

Sometimes agitation is so severe at mealtime that the person cannot be persuaded to eat. Ignore this and let them walk. Keep the meal warm, to be eaten when the person is calmer. Supervising the meal in the agitated person's room will often encourage eating, or it can be served with a friend in a nook away from the dining room.

## Slow eating and spilling

Slow eating and spilling are mostly due to the effects of the dementia illness or stroke damage which interferes or restricts the normal movement of arms and hands. Or it may be due to tremor associated with a neurological disorder such as Parkinson's disease. Heavy sedation can also interfere with normal eating to an extent where the person is unable to hold food in the mouth or swallow.

# Making a mess

The person who eats with their hands, drops food, slops it on the table or otherwise makes a mess is not aware of and not able to control what they are doing. Where this is likely, the person must not be left unsupervised. Scolding has no effect, except maybe to upset them.

# Disruptive behaviour

Disruptive behaviour—food throwing and sloppy and primitive eating—is distressing to others who are aware of it and those who retain their eating skills. They may be reluctant to come to the dining room or may leave before finishing the meal.

> Mrs Jason has lost a considerable amount of weight and her general health has deteriorated since coming to the nursing home. Her family is worried and seeks medical advice. She is suffering from malnutrition. She is more closely supervised by staff at mealtime.
>
> Mrs Jason's place at the table is next to two men who slop and drop food, and one whose food dribbles from his mouth. She has been in the habit of quietly, and unnoticed, leaving the table after only eating a few mouthfuls. When moved to another table, she again eats and her usual good health returns.

If this behaviour cannot be contained, seating the messy and disruptive eaters a little removed from the main body of residents, or apart in a cosy room where they can be supervised, will restore peace to the main dining room. When the need for segregation is over, they should return.

# Suggestions

◆ Serve one course of food at a time.
◆ Peel, core and seed fresh fruit. Remove bruised parts.
◆ Place jugs of water or juice, pepper and salt, butter, jams and sauces on a separate table or sideboard if they will be misused. Serve them as requested.

## Eating alone is not a good idea

Where meals are served at the bedside and the person is left alone, they often do not eat adequately. It is not uncommon for meals to be removed uneaten, often with plastic wrap intact or cover not removed. Or for the person to scrape food into a wastepaper basket or drawer; or for it to be pilfered by others.

Where individual supervision is not possible, provide a table where problem eaters can be supervised as a group.

## SEXUALITY AND SEXUAL BEHAVIOUR*

A person with dementia still has needs for love and affection, often of a sexual nature.

Sexual desires and fantasies may persist well into the illness.

Fears of sexual attack in a mixed unit are often unfounded. The anxiety is real.

Bathing and dressing will often arouse sexual desire.

Touching and hugging is usually appreciated, but may be misinterpreted.

Actions or conversations may be construed as having sexual overtones. Explain clearly what you are doing.

Sexual harassment is not to be tolerated.

Self-expressed intimacy, such as fondling and masturbating in public, needs to be contained.

Liaisons between residents may cause problems which need to be worked out with the family.

Sexuality encompasses a range of feelings and activities from the deepest longings for mutual affection to the simple enjoyment of the company of a loved one. It covers a gamut of behaviours—touching,

---

* For further reading, see this author's *Sex, Intimacy and Aged Care*, ACER Press, 1999

kissing, caressing and cuddling, genital intercourse with mutual orgasm and feelings of closeness and of being wanted and valued as a human being. There are two matters of concern in the area of sexuality in dementia care: first, meeting the need for affection, love and sexual gratification of the affected person; and second, sexually explicit behaviour, which creates problems for family carers, residents, staff and the person themself.

# Sexual desire

While some people lose interest in sexual activity quite early in the course of the dementia, others have a markedly increased hunger for sexual gratification. This may be due to a number of reasons: damage to the brain, prescription drugs, separation from the sexual partner, other external factors or the possibility that this is the only pleasure that the person has left. Consider also that the person may have always had a strong sexual drive and this for them is 'normal' behaviour.

Where a person has strong sexual desire that cannot be fulfilled, the consequence will certainly be frustration which will be manifested in behaviour, such as self-expressed intimacy— masturbating and self-fondling—and harassment of staff and other residents. This is discussed in more detail later in this section.

### *Meeting needs*

Many couples are engaged in a sexual relationship, despite the intervention of dementia, which is particularly satisfying to both. In many nursing homes and hostels the sexual needs of residents are largely ignored or placed low on the list of priorities of care.

When one or even both partners are moved to a residential facility, they may be deprived of opportunity for moments of intimacy and making love that they previously enjoyed. On the other hand, some facilities are sensitive to these needs and make provision for couples to have some privacy.

 The Masons are in their seventies. Up to the time Mr Mason is admitted to the nursing home, they enjoy a satisfactory sex life.

> Now he shares a room with three others. When Mrs Mason visits they walk together or sit beside his bed. Visitors are embarrassed and staff are disapproving when they come upon them in a passionate embrace. At times Mr Mason makes advances to female staff.
>
> Moving him into a single room gives the couple opportunities to be together undisturbed. Both are noticeably less stressed and Mr Mason's advances to female staff are now rare.

Even the opportunity to lie down together is comforting.

More difficult to accommodate are the needs for affection and an intimacy of the person who no longer has a partner. This person may form a liaison with another resident, gaining satisfaction from the companionship and affection associated with such a relationship.

## Sexual fantasies

Sexual fantasies are not uncommon in people affected by dementia.

> Mrs White, 79 years old and mother of eight, happily relives her child-bearing days. She fantasises sexual intercourse with an 80-year-old resident, and a resulting pregnancy. Placing the nurse's hand on her distended abdomen, she says, 'Feel baby. Feel baby.'
>
> Her face lights up when a nurse takes a moment or two to talk to her about her 'baby'. When people do not understand and recoil in embarrassment, she stands confused, with tears trickling down her face.
>
> ———
>
> Judging from the way John is acting, it seems certain he believes the ward is a brothel. Although he has little speech, his demands for sexual gratification are clear. When no male attendant is available at bath time, female staff have difficulty controlling him.
>
> According to his wife, John is a virtuous man, a loyal husband and devoted to his daughter. Using this information, one young nurse finds a way to control him. 'Please, John, stop. Just think of me as your daughter.'

# Sexual fears

Fears of sexual attack are not unusual where residents are mobile and genders mixed. Residents who undress in public or who wander partly clothed are viewed by others as a sexual threat. Female residents in particular feel intimidated by aggressive male residents wandering into their rooms to lie on the bed.

Usually fears are unfounded—the wanderer, prompted by the sight of the bed enters the room to lie down. However the anxiety and fear are real. Deal with them by personal or group discussion. Explain your own difficulty in dealing with strippers or wanderers and assure residents of their safety.

### *Apprehensive of staff*

Embarrassment at being undressed and showered by a stranger, especially a member of the opposite sex, may arouse anxiety and the person may resist. Very often this reaction is at times associated with the older generation's strong attitude of modesty. Using force or insisting will not improve the situation and may provoke a violent reaction.

If the problem persists, the home carer or a member of the family could be asked to be present at bath time for a few times. Choose a time convenient to the family. On page 98 we discussed the case of Mrs Prim and how her resistance to showering was overcome.

# The wrong message

Sometimes a person's strange and disruptive behaviour emanates from their misunderstanding of a care worker's actions and words. For example, the man being showered by a female nurse may interpret this as having a sexual meaning. Words can also be misinterpreted.

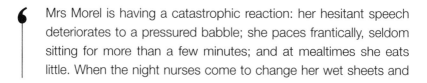

Mrs Morel is having a catastrophic reaction: her hesitant speech deteriorates to a pressured babble; she paces frantically, seldom sitting for more than a few minutes; and at mealtimes she eats little. When the night nurses come to change her wet sheets and nightdress, she is fully dressed, lying on top of the bedclothes. She screams and struggles when they undress her, and on the next round they find her fully dressed again.

Finally we piece together what is troubling her. When the night nurses wake her from her drugged sleep to change her, she demands, 'Why are you doing this?' They soothe her, 'Because we love you.' Her confused mind tells her that the only reason these young women 'love' her is for some sexual purpose.

Mrs Morel's terror subsides when the nurses tell her: 'We are changing your sheets and nightie because you are wet. You will be more comfortable.'

## *Touching*

Cuddling and hugging are usually welcomed and appreciated. Occasionally, though, these advances are misinterpreted.

# Sexually explicit behaviour

It is not unusual for a person with dementia to engage in some type of sexually explicit activity. This behaviour does not always have a sexual motive, but may have a number of other triggers.

## *Masturbation and self-fondling*

For obvious reasons these two activities are called 'self-expressed intimacy'. Occasionally when a person's sense of social control is diminished, he or she will masturbate or engage in genital fondling in a public place, often causing embarrassment and distress to other people.

Mocking and scolding is not an option to contain this behaviour and may distress the person unnecessarily. An effective way to handle this behaviour is to quietly remove the person to the privacy of their own room or other unfrequented area.

This behaviour may be habitual—the way that the person has always relieved sexual tension and obtained sexual gratification. On the other hand it may have nothing whatever to do with sex. Reasons for a person masturbating can be a reaction to the discomfort of tight clothing or temperature that is too high, urgency to relieve the bladder or bowel or even boredom. All of these will act as triggers for the behaviour.

## Public exposure

This often takes the form of a person appearing partly undressed in a public place, such as the dining room in a nursing home or hostel, or walking into the front garden or street at home.

Someone may even undress in public. In the majority of cases, this sort of behaviour has a simple explanation. Dressing and undressing is a pretty normal behaviour; we all dress and undress at least once every day. It is the place that is incongruous; the person with dementia has simply lost the ability to recognise that it is not appropriate to undress in a public place. Discomfort, boredom and distress would need to be taken into account as the reason for shedding garments.

Quietly remove the person to their own room and help them to fully clothe themselves.

> Mrs C. was distressed for several days after being transferred from hospital to a dementia unit. One night she was missing. They found her in the garden. Her clothes were neatly folded on the garden bench and she was dancing, whirling and swaying with great energy. Stark naked. Night staff covered her in a blanket, brought her in and gave her a warm drink. On putting her to bed, one of them stayed with her until she fell asleep.

Occasionally someone will deliberately expose their genital area, but not always with sexual intent.

## Urinating in public places

Urinating in public is usually associated with the person no longer being able to find the way to the toilet. Sometimes it is also triggered by discomfort. A receptacle such as a bucket or wastepaper basket can be mistaken for a toilet and so stimulate the person, often a man, to urinate. Regular toileting is effective in some instances of spontaneous urination.

While sexually explicit behaviours, especially those of self-expressed intimacy, are considered to be sexually motivated, they are often due to some other reason. And while a person usually does not behave in this way with the intention of harassing others, there are instances when the behaviour is thought to be deliberate and, on occasions, in retaliation for a perceived wrong.

## Sexual harassment

One of the most difficult of behaviours with sexual overtones to deal with is harassment. Staff of residential facilities in particular are targets for the person who sexually harasses; residents also can be at risk. A favourite ploy of the harasser is to corner a care worker in the shower, while another is to expose himself in front of young staff. Obscene language and 'touching' are other common harassing techniques. It is not unusual for the home carer to be the victim of sexual harassment, often having to submit under force to the harasser.

Regardless of whether the harasser is aware that their behaviour is inappropriate, it cannot be allowed to continue. Action should be taken to assess the problem situation and contain the behaviour without delay.

# LOSS AND GRIEF

**The person with dementia experiences loss and suffers grief as we all do.**

**The grief is real even though it may be associated with something that happened a long time ago.**

**Sometimes the grief is overwhelming and sometimes fleeting.**

**Do not ignore grief; sympathise with the feelings.**

**Let the person know it is all right to be sad.**

**Death of a family member or close friend must be handled.**

# Dealing with loss and grief

At some time in our lives we suffer a loss: a broken romance, divorce, moving house and leaving friends, older children leaving home or the death of a loved one. We feel sad, we grieve.

For many of us, dealing with someone else's grief is difficult. We feel helpless and do not know what to say. Sometimes it makes us feel better if we try to cheer them up. Sometimes we avoid them. When people grieve, they need to experience a range of emotions. To recognise and respond to these feelings and convey 'It's OK to be sad' helps someone come to terms with the grief. If you are able to say a simple 'I'm sorry', it conveys to the grieving person that you care.

# Dementing people grieve

A person with dementia can experience loss, and grieve as we all do. Some may grieve for their lost life, a role or a skill that no longer exists. For some it is an overwhelming emotion; for others it is fleeting and can be easily distracted.

### Grieving for long ago

It may be difficult to understand when deep grief is associated with a loss experienced a long time ago. This grief is as real as the grief for a recent loss. For that person, it is happening here and now.

> Fifty-nine years old and widowed, Helen lives with her daughter Nancy and her family until she comes to the nursing home. Helen is overwhelmed by grief. 'Where's Nancy? ... I want Nancy,' she sobs. Assurances that Nancy will come are met with a choked, 'No, she won't come. She's dead. I'll never see her again.'
>
> The sudden separation from Nancy revives the trauma of the disappearance of her younger daughter, Pat, when she was twenty. Helen's confused mind mixes up the two daughters and she is anxious for both, grieving both. Occasionally her fears can be soothed by our putting our arms around her and sympathising, 'It's terrible what happened to Pat, but Nancy is coming to see you today.'

Sometimes she can be distracted by our walking with her in the garden or holding her hand and saying, 'Tell me about your grandson Paul.' When she is distraught to the point of frenzy, only a telephone call to Nancy convinces her that her daughter is alive.

### Grieving for the here and now

Sometimes the grief is associated with something that is currently happening. It is not unusual for a person to grieve for the losses associated with dementia.

'It's awful to be old and lose your memory,' Ivy repeats to everyone around her. Ivy's grief is fleeting. Ninety years of age, with beautiful old-world manners, she showers and dresses herself and knits in a purl one, drop one fashion. She does not remember the location of her room and introduces her son, 'I think this is my father.'

'I come from Brisbane ... I think I come from Brisbane ... y'know my memory isn't good these days,' she says, the tears welling up. 'It's awful to be old and lose your memory. I hate being old.'

Her grief soon passes when we comfort her, 'You feel pretty sad because you forget.' A kiss and a cuddle and she takes up her knitting or chats to the women sitting beside her.

## Handling death

Sometimes a family member will undertake to break the news to a relative, while some will pass the responsibility to the staff of a residential facility. Where the dead person is the only close support of the resident, staff have no alternative but to handle the situation. To get some indication of how the person will react to the news, always tell them of the death.

### Different reactions

There is no one way that people with dementia react to the news of a death. It is essential that you accept and go along with the individual way that a person with dementia handles a death and not expect them to conform to some proscribed pattern of grieving. Some will fully understand and go through the full process of grieving and will need to have your full support during this time. Others will understand and seem to forget almost immediately while some will reject the news, and react with loud distress.

## Denying the death

'Max and Freda were children of the Holocaust. They were the only two of their family to survive and both lived in the same nursing home. When Freda was moved to a dementia hostel, Max still spent his days with her. The day after Max died, staff gently told Freda: 'Darling, we have some sad news for you, your brother Max died last night.' 'Not dead, not dead!' screeched Freda, as she rushed from her room. They tried for a day or two to tell Freda that Max would not be coming any more because he had died, only to receive the same reaction. In between times, she would wander through the unit, looking for Max and crying his name.

Without mentioning Max's death again, staff gave Freda considerable sympathy and support and recognised her sadness by simply saying 'You are sad about Max', or 'You miss Max'. Her grief gradually dissipated. '

## Replacing the dead person

Sometimes the person with dementia will handle the death of a loved one by replacing them with another.

'Mrs Younger lived at home with her husband Roy, who had cared for her ever since she was diagnosed with Alzheimer's disease, until Roy died. She did not seem to comprehend that he had died, nor did she exhibit any distress, immediately 'adopting' her son-in-law as her husband.

Within days she was moved into a nursing home, where they insisted that she must come to terms with her husband's death, constantly telling her that Roy was dead. They instructed the son-in-law not to visit until Mrs Younger had 'accepted' Roy's death.

Mrs Younger gradually became more despondent and aggressive and spiteful to other residents, and at times physically violent with staff. She was sedated to control the disruptive behaviour.

Eventually the family found alternative accommodation in a specialised dementia unit, where staff were quite agreeable for the son-in-law to visit. Mrs Younger was content and sedation was discontinued.

### *It is better to tell*

If told immediately or shortly after it occurs, many people with dementia seem to be able to handle a death in the family fairly well. Some will grieve for a day or two, or from time to time, but will eventually come to terms with the death, in their own way.

However if a long period elapses between the death and the time of telling, particularly if the death is of a close relation, you may notice a growing anxiety at the dead person's absence. In these circumstances, the delayed telling will sometimes arouse disbelief, anger or chronic withdrawal.

When a death is imminent, it is better to mention it occasionally, so that the person becomes used to the notion of death. However, do not emphasise the impending death so as to provoke the person to react adversely. The same procedure can be followed when a resident in the unit dies or is dying.

Catastrophic reactions are not uncommon as a reaction to the death of a close relative, or even a popular resident.

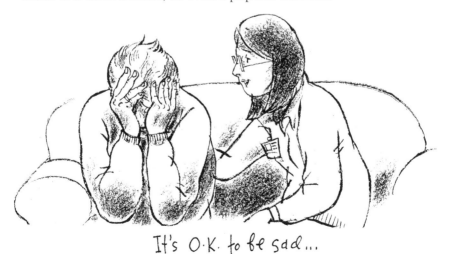

It's O.K. to be sad...

# CHAPTER EIGHT

# Worker skills

## COMMUNICATING *

Communication with others is achieved by our sending messages and responding to the messages we receive.

To help the person with dementia to understand you, keep your message simple and back up your words with body language.

Allow for communication barriers and impaired sight and hearing.

Wait for a response. It may take some time for the person's brain to process what you say.

If you have difficulty in understanding the person with dementia, try to pick up clues: a single word, an action or a facial expression.

Listen for the message beneath the words, and listen for the feeling. Let the person know you have understood by reflecting the words and feeling tone.

## Interpersonal communication

Think of interpersonal communication as:

◆ sending messages
◆ receiving messages
◆ responding to messages—face to face with another person

Our needs and wishes, our ideas and feelings are communicated to others by sending messages and responding to the messages we receive.

*Read this section in conjunction with 'Misunderstandings and misusing words' Chapter 3.

We do this by:

◆  speaking and writing words
◆  hearing and reading
◆  our attitude and mood
◆  our body language and facial expressions (a smile, a frown),
   actions and gestures: the way we sit, stand and move sends a
   message
◆  our tone of voice
◆  pictures and graphics

## Communication difficulties

The type of communication problems that are associated with
dementia vary from person to person, depending on the stage and
type of illness, and the degree and nature of the brain impairment.

### *Impaired sight and hearing*

Many elderly people are cut off from satisfactory communication
because their sight and hearing are impaired. Make sure the person
can see and hear you.

◆  Use the person's name and identify yourself.
◆  Touch them lightly on the arm and hand to attract attention.
◆  Stand and sit so that your face is level with theirs and the
   movement of your lips is easily seen.
◆  Speak slowly and clearly but do not shout.
◆  You may have to repeat your message several times.

### *Other barriers to communication*

All of our day-to-day communication is filtered or screened
through the influence of our personal life experiences, our moods
and our beliefs which bias what we say to others and the way we
say it. When we listen to the world around us and to the people
in our lives, what we hear is also interpreted through our filters.
The individual differences in our filters can often account for the
fact that the message sent is not the message that is received. A

person who has emigrated from a tribal home in Africa will have filters different from one who has been raised in middle class western culture.

A simple example of the way that our filters bias what we say and what we hear is the old childhood game in which the first person in the circle tells a story, and as the story travels around the circle, it is subtly changed as it passes through each teller's filters.

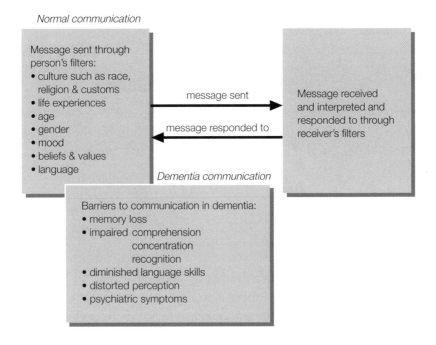

The person with dementia will retain their filters for some time into the course of the condition but what they say and what they hear is also affected by another layer of filters, which we call barriers and which contribute to difficulties in understanding others and being understood. Speech and language impairment, diminished comprehension and memory, short attention span, hallucinations, delusions and so on will act as barriers to communication for the person with dementia. Even a simple message such as 'Eve, please put the book down' cannot be understood by the person who no longer knows what a book looks like or where 'down' is.

# Making yourself understood

The person with dementia may become frustrated, angry or apathetic if the brain is not making sense of what you are saying. You can help understanding by:

- using simple language
- using body language—gestures, actions and facial expressions
- showing
- breaking the message into parts

### Communicating with words

If the person still has some understanding of words, use single, short, simple and specific sentences:

- 'Norma, please come to lunch.'
- 'John, you look smart in your red jumper.'
- 'Helen, would you like to come for a walk?'
- 'Mrs Simpson, your daughter Julie is coming to see you.'

These communications:

- attract attention by first using the person's name
- are simple and short
- are specific—have one definite message
- use a single sentence
- are not difficult to understand

### What not to do

*Communication 1* 'We're going for a bus trip, after you've had morning tea and I've taken you to the toilet. If you like you can watch TV while you're waiting. Oh no . . . it might be easier to just sit there and talk to Jim until we're ready.'

In this communication, the messages keep changing. The dementing listener, unable to hop from idea to idea, picks up only one message or none at all, and probably becomes confused and reacts with irritation or withdrawal.

*Communication 2* 'What's the matter? Can't you see I'm busy? If you'll only try to tell me what's wrong I might be able to do something about it. Gosh, where are your shoes? You've only got one shoe on and only one stocking, I don't know...'

The feeling underlying this message is unmistakable. The listener may not make sense of all the words, but they will certainly get the message that they are a nuisance and the sender is impatient. Both these communications are unsatisfactory because they are complex: too many ideas and too many messages.

### *Body language*

Your facial expression, body posture, gestures, tone of voice as well as words all send messages. Of these, facial expressions is the most important—even in normal conversation facial expression has the greatest impact, followed by tone of voice (pleasant but not patronising), and lastly words. If the person has difficulty in understanding words, make it more possible for them to receive the message you intend to convey: your body language and words should send the same message. If the messages conflict, then the message received will be unclear or incorrect. For instance, if your message is 'It's nearly bedtime' but your voice is harsh and your facial expression stern, the message received will most probably tell the listener that you are displeased, and they will react accordingly.

You will be surprised how quickly it becomes commonplace for you to use facial expressions, actions and gestures to back up your words, and how much more easily you are understood.

◆ 'James, would you like a drink?' Look at him, tilt your head and raise your eyebrows slightly, holding the cup or glass so that he can see it.
◆ 'Mrs Goode, time for bed.' Close your eyes and put your head on the side, resting on your hands.
◆ 'Mr Jackson, please don't do that.' Frown and shake your head.
◆ 'Ssshh.' Put your finger across your lips.
◆ 'Josh, come for a walk?' Hold out your hand, palm upwards or cup his elbow.
◆ 'Lunchtime now.' Chewing movements and spooning actions reinforce this message.

## *Show*

Showing as well as telling helps you get the message across.

> Mrs Moore cannot comprehend 'Go the toilet now', even when she is taken to the bathroom. If the nurse arranges her clothes in readiness and points to the toilet, she remembers what to do. She is praised. After completing her toilet, she stands up, rearranges her clothing, smiles at the nurse and says, 'OK now.'
>
> ———
>
> 'Throw the ball, Frank,' the group around the circle choruses as they reach out with cupped hands. The diversional therapist repeatedly places the large soft ball in his hands, raising his arms in throwing movements. Sometimes the ball lies where it rolls into Frank's lap and sometimes it drops to the floor. Then one day a glimmer of memory surfaces; his face opens in a toothy grin. As the ball comes towards him, Frank raises his foot—and kicks it!

## *Break the message into parts*

Sometimes the brain cannot understand concepts such as 'Get dressed', 'Get on the bus' or 'Come to the dining room.'

Try something like this:

1 'Pat, we're going to the dining room now.'
2 'Stand up', holding out your hand ready to assist in case she does not understand.
3 'Hold my arm', looping your arm through hers.
4 'Now we're going to turn this way', slowly changing direction.
5 'That's good.'
6 'Now we'll walk.'

This example breaks the message up into small parts. Words are backed up by facial expression, gestures and actions to help Pat understand.

# Asking questions

Questions can sometimes be great starters for social interaction. When giving simple choices it is better to use questions that need 'yes' or 'no' answers, but be prepared for the person not to understand what it is you are asking.

◆ 'Bert, would you like a piece of cake?'
◆ 'Mr Fry, would you like to sit outside?'

This is more easily understood than questions with multiple choices, such as ' …cake, biscuit or sandwich?' or '…outside or in the sitting room?'

When you need information, it is quicker for you and easier for the person to comprehend if you ask a question that requires a yes/no answer.

◆ 'Mrs Pringle, is your foot hurting?', touching foot.
◆ 'Joseph, do you have a sore throat?', frown and point to throat.

## *Be cautious*

As a general rule, caution needs to be exercised when questioning the person with dementia. Sometimes, probing for information or asking too many questions will trigger a negative reaction. Some people will confabulate, or patiently answer our questions in order to please us. On other occasions, resentment at an unwanted intrusion into their privacy may be verbalised.

We at least need to be aware of what our objective is in asking the question. What is the purpose of the question? Trying to reawaken memory? Probing out of curiosity? Are we trying to stimulate social interaction?

Questions such as 'Do you remember what you did this morning?' or 'Do you know who this lady is?' may increase confusion or cause panic. If the person does not remember, they may answer 'Yes' or 'Of course I do', but burst into tears or gaze into space. Turn these sorts of questions around: 'We did . . . this morning' and 'Here is your wife come to see you.'

# Statements initiate discussion

A statement will usually elicit an interested response and stimulate discussion, and is less likely to result in an undesirable reaction.

◆ 'Some of us like to watch football on Saturday.'
◆ 'We all enjoyed the barbecue at lunchtime.'
◆ 'Mrs Cartwright's daughter brought a lovely bunch of flowers.'

# Wait for a response

Do you recall the story on p. 59 about the student and the man who took days to respond to her questions?

The failing brain often takes time to process a message. A blank stare may not mean that someone does not comprehend. The brain may be slow in processing what you have said. Wait. It may take several minutes for the person to give you an answer.

If after waiting you do not receive a response, repeat or rephrase your message. This will sometimes have the desired effect. On rare occasions you may be approached hours or days later with a response. Recognise this and praise the person by saying: 'Thank you for telling me. It's good that you remembered!'

# Listening and hearing

When someone is trying to tell or ask you something, listen.

> The nurse coming on duty smiles when she hears Peter tell his wife he has just had a bad fall. 'Now then, Peter, none of your tales. He's always imagining something or other', she explains to his wife.
>
> Peter's face flushes and contorts and words tumble over words, as his hands clutch the air attempting to point to the gash on the back of his head.

### Hear the underlying message

There are times, however, when listening to the words is not enough. You need to hear what the person is telling you *beneath* the words.

The woman who says 'My daughter is taking me home tomorrow' and the man packing his suitcase are both telling you they do not want to be here. Do not respond by saying: 'This is your home now' or 'Let's unpack your case, you're not going anywhere'. This will cause greater feelings of helplessness and anxiety.

Respond to the message underneath by saying: 'It's frightening being in a strange place' or 'You're missing your home? I would be sad too'. Then reassure the person and divert his attention: 'Your wife will be here soon. Let's go and get your new shirt on.'

# Picking up clues

It is harder to hear the message when the person cannot communicate thoughts clearly and when speech is garbled, limited or otherwise does not make sense. Then you have to rely on picking up clues. The clue may be a word, an emotion, a gesture or an expression that indicates what the person is trying to tell you.

With practice and patience, and when you get to know the person better, you will become sensitive to clues.

## *Word clues*

' When Gerald demands of staff 'Want one, want one', they know he is asking for a cigarette.

———

Mavis asks, 'Please money...you know, doesn't live here any... want thing...you know, sick.' The personal care assistant knows what is bothering her and answers, 'You're worried that your husband might be sick? I'm sure he's all right, but we'll telephone him anyway.'

———

At the day centre every afternoon at three o'clock, Mrs Smith clutches the recreation worker: '...getting late...oh...something or thing...lamb chops...tidy up...', expressing a number of incomplete ideas, all related to home. She is reassured by the response: 'You'll be going home soon.' '

### *Wordless clues*

Wordless clues may be given by the person to emphasise the message. Even the person who is no longer able to find words may give clear non-verbal clues. By observing the person's characteristic way of communicating you will become sensitive to these clues. You will automatically respond to:

◆ a frown—'Harry, something's bothering you. Tell me about it.'
◆ tears—'Aahh, you're upset. Sit down and we'll talk about it.'
◆ a grimace—'You don't like your dinner? I'll bring you some sandwiches.'
◆ a smile—'That's a lovely smile. You look happy.'

Increased agitation, removal of clothing and a flushed face may indicate a need to go to the toilet. Wandering back and forth to the dining room may indicate that the person is hungry.

Mr Allen has had no speech since his last stroke. He can indicate most of his needs and converse with staff using actions and gestures.

―――――

Claire wordlessly holds up the presents her daughter brought. Her face lights in a beautiful smile when we admire them.

## Symbolism

Sometimes a person with dementia will use symbols when talking to you. Symbolism is the substitution of an idea for another idea. On p. 137 I wrote about Mrs Morel. Staff had great difficulty in understanding Mrs Morel, but one of the clues that led us to the solution of the problem was her use of word symbolism. We noticed that she repeatedly referred to 'the mother and the daughter', 'niece and aunty', 'the grown-up and the child'. We eventually guessed that she was referring to the two night nurses who attended to her. One of the nurses was quite tiny, while the other was nearly 180 centimetres tall. Mrs Morel had been using these phrases as symbols for 'short and tall' or 'big and little'.

> Then there is Sylvia, who is becoming frustrated at her inability to convey to the recreation worker how she is feeling right now. She leads her to the young pine tree in the hostel garden. Stretching her arms around the trunk, she says 'Feel life, alive—strong, strong', and touches her chest and shakes her head. The worker replies, 'I hear you telling me you feel all dead inside', as tears well in Sylvia's eyes. She has been understood.

The person who likes to paint and draw may indicate a feeling or memory through symbolism in their art.

### A very obscure message

> Living in a unit for elderly Jewish people, Mrs Jamison can pursue the customs of her religion. Her comprehension is fair but she is often frustrated at her inability to communicate, even though she knows what she wants to say.
>
> One afternoon in the recreation room she shows signs of increasing agitation, grumbles and makes aggressive movements towards the man sitting opposite her at the craft table. Holding her hand and speaking quietly, we piece together the clues, checking each one with Mrs Jamison. We know Mrs Jamison has a healthy appetite; the table where she sits is the same as those in the dining room. Her poking movements towards the man's head indicate her distress because he is not wearing his skullcap at the 'dining table'. He agrees to put on the skullcap. Still agitated, she shakes her head. Finally we ask, 'Are you hungry?' She smiles and nods.
>
> 'You will have a cup of tea and cake soon. It's almost afternoon teatime.' She relaxes.

# Reflecting

'Reflecting' is a word used to describe the mirror imaging of what you believe the person is telling you with their words, emotions and body language. Reflecting is one of the most valuable interpersonal communication skills. As well as confirming that you have heard the correct message, it may also act as a prompt, helping the person to express the message more clearly. Reflecting is also effective in that it tells the person you have understood, and so has a positive effect on self-esteem.

## *Reflecting feelings*

The recreation worker we spoke of earlier reflected Sylvia's feelings of devastation about the ravages of her dementia by picking up the clues in both her words and actions, although most emotions are more easily identified than in that example. In that incident, Sylvia's true feelings were difficult to recognise because they were disguised by symbolism. Sometimes an occasional word such as 'death', 'sick', 'alone', 'home', or 'funny' will give you a clue to what the person is feeling. Emotions are also expressed non-verbally, by facial expression and body posture: the person sitting alone and slumped is probably feeling sad or rejected. Respond to that message too, by reflecting his feelings: 'You seem to be lonely sitting here.'

You do not always have to use words to reflect the message; a hug, a squeeze of the hand or your facial expression will often more adequately reflect the feeling.

---

**As dementia worsens, a person will communicate less with words and more with feelings.**
**Emotions and behaviour may be the only way that someone can communicate with you.**

---

## *Reflecting words*

The person with dementia may substitute a similar-sounding word, describe a word, use single words or speak in disjointed phrases. On most occasions, if you focus your listening and observe all the clues, you will be able to make an educated guess as to the meaning of the message. For example, the woman points to the radio:

Woman: 'I think . . . I want . . . know everything that's going on.'
Carer: 'You want to listen to the news?'
Woman: 'Yes, I want to hear the news.'

Wherever dialogue has been used throughout this book, you will find a number of examples where reflecting has been used.

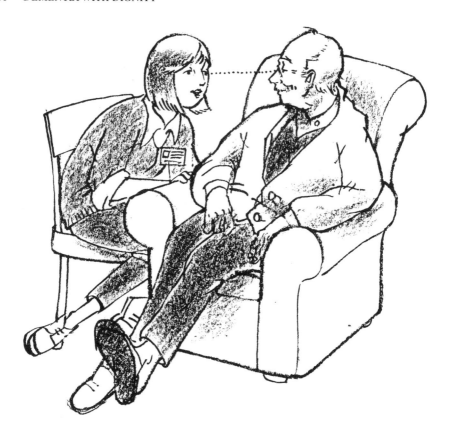

## Speaking a different language

A language acquired later in life is usually lost before the person's native language. Usually the person uses snatches of both the first and the acquired languages, but eventually makes sense in neither. In such circumstances, interpreting the words is of little use.

It is not unusual in a nursing home or day centre where there are people of several different cultures to find a group of people, none of whom speak the same language, happily 'chatting' to each other. Some may have even lost the use of words, yet they communicate with smiles, nods and other social devices that are habitual to them.

To help you to communicate with people you do not understand, and where the person still has some word comprehension, compile a list of significant words in that language, such as 'toilet', 'eat', 'come', and so on. Where understanding is limited, as with everyone, you will have to rely on body language. When possible, employing staff and volunteers from the same cultural backgrounds as the residents is of great assistance.

## GUIDELINES FOR INTERPERSONAL COMMUNICATION

◆ Sit, stand or kneel so that you have level eye contact.

◆ Use the person's name and identify yourself.

◆ Touch gently, where appropriate.

◆ Speak slowly and clearly. Use short, simple sentences.

◆ Use body language and facial expression.

◆ Match words, body language and facial expression.

◆ Communicate understanding attitudes.

◆ Focus your listening. Pick up a word or an expression you can respond to.

◆ Respond to feelings.

◆ Pick up on symbolism.

◆ Reflect the message you hear and prompt if appropriate.

◆ Be patient. Wait for a response.

# THE WORKING RELATIONSHIP

A working relationship is a very special relationship, built on trust and empathy.

There are several differences between a working relationship and a personal relationship.

Ending a working relationship in an appropriate way will ease the separation for both the client and the worker.

Your part of the relationship with the person with dementia is demonstrated by your warm, caring attitude.

# Understanding relationship

When we use the word 'relationship' in this sense, we mean the feelings between two people that affect the way they behave towards each other.

# The working relationship

A good working relationship is the basis for everything we do with and for our client, whether it be the person with dementia or the carer, or others who seek our assistance.

## *A very special sort of relationship*

In dementia care, a working relationship is the type and quality of our interaction with the person with dementia, the family and our colleagues that:

♦ allows us to achieve our goals for that person with dementia;
♦ supports kinship relationships.

When we establish a good working relationship, our client will trust us. Feelings of safety and the self-esteem of the person with dementia will be enhanced and carers will have confidence that we are competent to do the job they expect us to do.

As well as trust, a good working relationship is built on empathy, that is, understanding the circumstances, reactions and feelings of the person we are working with as though they were our own—a sort of stepping into the other person's shoes.

## *A different sort of relationship*

If we are to provide our client with the best possible service, we need to be aware of the differences between a working relationship and a personal relationship. Otherwise we may find ourselves stepping across the fine line that separates the provider of a friendly, understanding service from a personal relationship.

Of course there are obvious differences: a working relationship is associated with our employment, paid or voluntary, to do a specific job of work, and being accountable to our employer and our client to carry out that work to the best of our ability. As well, a working relationship does not have the emotional ties or entanglements of a personal relationship.

Sometimes residential staff and respite workers* in the home, more so than workers who see their clients occasionally, can find themselves almost moving into the role of the home carer, and the home carer, particularly a spouse, can feel pushed aside. This happens because the worker's contact tends to continue over a long period and involves intimate bodily caring, as well as being called on to meet the emotional needs of the person with dementia—a very close, caring relationship.

Another major difference is that, unlike a personal relationship, a working relationship has a planned beginning and a foreseeable end. It does not carry on after the job is done.

> In the agency for which she works, Sarah Smith is a highly sought-after respite worker. She forms a deep attachment to 'my people' and if and when they are transferred to a nursing home or dementia hostel, she makes weekly visits to each one, taking meals to some and discussing their wellbeing with staff. The outcome in this instance is:
>
> 1   Staff of the facility relate more to Sarah then they do to the family, a fact which the home carer resents.
>
> 2   Professional workers find that their work is impeded by Sarah's close relationship to the resident and, on occasions, her interference.
>
> 3   Sarah herself becomes overburdened with looking after 'my people' and has little time for her respite work. Eventually she gives up the visiting, leaving a difficult situation for others to resolve.

## Ending the relationship

Your client may be the person with dementia; it may be the family care giver. Whoever it is there can be any number of reasons for

---

*I have used the term 'worker' to refer to any person who is employed to work in the area of dementia care, regardless of thier discipline or training.

ending a working relationship: the person you have been caring for at home or at the day centre may be moving to a nursing home or hostel; the family may be moving away from the district; the person may have been referred to another service more appropriate to their needs; you might be leaving, or changing your job at your workplace and another worker is taking over.

Whatever the reason, we should aim to terminate the relationship with the client in a way that makes it as easy as possible for both the client and ourselves. We also want clients to feel comfortable about coming back to our service should they need us in the future. There are certain procedures for ending a working relationship satisfactorily. Here are some suggestions that you might find useful.

1   As soon as you are aware of the change, discuss it with your client and talk about it as often as your client feels is necessary. Include the person with dementia in your discussion. If your daily work is with the dementing person, mention it occasionally, but not so often as to increase anxiety.

2   Support the person through the transfer. There is invariably some anxiety around the separation, especially if the relationship has been a satisfactory one over a long period. As well as apprehension about leaving the old service and experiencing feelings of insecurity about the new service, the carer will also feel sad about leaving a worker she has come to rely on. Encourage the carer to confide these feelings in you and share your own feelings about the parting.

3   There are some practical ways you can ease the transfer: arrange a visit to the new agency or facility; introduce staff; introduce the new worker—maybe a joint interview if appropriate. In case of a move from the district, obtain as much information as you can about services available in the new district, or arrange for pamphlets to be forwarded to your client. Better still, arrange a personal meeting with a worker who might act as a resource person or key worker until the client finds their way around in the new network. Put them in touch with the local carers' group.

4   Make one follow-up contact to ensure that the client has received the appropriate services and that there are no major problems. It is not advisable to maintain a continuing contact. If you do so, it

will be more difficult for a new worker to make a satisfactory relationship with the client, and this will to some extent affect the quality of service the carer and person with dementia will receive.

5   If you are still working with the client and the person with dementia dies, the carer may want to continue her contact with you for some time. It is important for the carer that you agree to this. By allowing them to maintain contact with you, you are offering an avenue of support from someone who has shared some of their most difficult and vulnerable times, and understands, probably better than anyone else, how they are feeling. She will move on when she is ready.

6   Don't forget *yourself*. Deal with your own anxiety at the separation; unburden to a colleague.

## Relating to the person with dementia

In working with people with dementia, the worker's part of the relationship is demonstrated by a warm, caring attitude. People who are affected by dementia are sensitive to attitudes and will quickly pick up our feelings towards them. They respond to our concern for their wellbeing, trust us and cooperate, thus making our work easier and more satisfying. You will find the relationship easier if you:

◆   develop caring attitudes, based on knowledge and understanding of the dementing process;
◆   avoid inappropriate attitudes and prejudices that result from ignorance and false beliefs;
◆   treat the person with dementia as an adult individual;
◆   be patient, interested and understanding—do not patronise;
◆   consider and respond to the person's feelings;
◆   develop the skill to step into the strange, confused world of the person with dementia.

### *You begin the relationship*

Because the person with dementia has most likely lost the capacity to initiate relationships, it is our responsibility to begin and maintain the contact.

## *No time for a relationship?*

Your shifts change frequently? You are only relieving? You're not going to be with the person long enough for a relationship to grow?

Even though relationships grow and strengthen over time, all relationships begin the moment you say 'Hello'.

---

**People with dementia may forget your name or where you fit into their lives, but they will invariably remember and respond to the satisfying relationship they have with you.**

---

# STEPPING INTO THE PERSON'S WORLD

---

**As dementia worsens, the affected person lives more and more in their own strange, confused or distorted world.**

**Attempting to convince the person of the 'real' world as we see it may only result in further confusion and, in many instances, some distress.**

**We need to develop the very special skill of being able to step into the personal world of the person with dementia.**

**In this section we discuss several 'worlds' of the person with dementia: including a past world, delusional and hallucinatory worlds, a world of confabulation and a distorted world.**

---

Throughout this book, you will find many examples of how workers and family carers were able to relate and communicate, and even solve problems, by stepping into the confused and often distorted world of the person with dementia. One example is the anecdote about Mr Adams in Chapter 5.

As dementia diseases progress, the grasp of the 'real' world slips away, and the private world of the affected person exists only in their mind. To work effectively with people affected by dementia, we need to understand this and learn to respond to the person's own strange, private world. If we try to convince the person that our world is the only real world, and that they are wrong, they will usually become more confused and may be overtly distressed, or may switch off, fixing us with a bewildered look. We are telling them one thing—our reality—and their brain is telling them another—their reality.

# A world of the past

Living in the past, or more properly living in the present as though it is the past, is probably the most frequently encountered 'other world' of the person with dementia. In a residential facility, there is the woman who intermittently worries about her children coming home from school, or another who talks about having to go home to look after her mother. Step into that world; treat it as real and respond to the person accordingly. If the anxiety persists, you may have to use a diversionary tactic, such as offering a cup of tea of involving the person in an activity.

> For forty years, Mr Jimson had been a taxi driver. He talks about his cab and his mates as though his past life still exists. He moves from that topic to tell anecdotes of his life in the country when he was a boy, and believes he still lives there with his grandfather.
>
> Sometimes he is anxious about forgetting where he parked the green Ford he owned a long time ago.
>
> Hostel staff step into his world. They encourage him to talk about his past experiences; they provide opportunities for him to wash a car belonging to one of the staff, an activity he enjoys. Sometimes they accompany him to the car park while he looks for his green car, and when he can't find it, they suggest that it might be at the service station being repaired. He seems satisfied with this explanation, and these activities fill most of his waking hours.

# A delusional world

Sometimes delusions will pervade most of a person's life:

> Heidi loved the somewhat tattered celluloid doll. She rocked it and she bathed it, dressed and undressed it, fed it and burped it,

wrapped it in a bunny rug and kissed it, and laid it down and happily sang it to sleep—several times a day. Staff would sometimes help her look after 'Baby', and even though she seemed to have difficulty understanding most things, pride would overcome her when they admired the doll.

New administration at the nursing home did not allow residents to have dolls, on the grounds that it projected the image of dementing people as children. 'Baby' had to go. Heidi became irritable, aggressive and at times morose and reluctant to eat. She appeared to be grieving. A photograph shows a disconsolate old woman slumped in a chair, uninterested in the activity of residents around her.

On p. 143 we discussed Mrs Younger who happily lived with the delusion that her son-in-law was her dead husband. The delusion pervaded all her waking hours.

# A hallucinatory world

Edward 'sees things'. He imagines a snarling face on the broom standing in the corner. Sometimes he is so frightened that he hides under the bed or behind a door.

Both his wife and the respite worker who comes to stay with him treat his terror as real. They step into his world. They sympathise with his fear and assure him that they will protect him; he will be safe with them. Sometimes they will challenge the 'monster' and order it out of the house. One day when his wife was out, he saw a monster coming through the door—it was the respite worker. Quickly, the respite worker removed his baseball cap and said to Edward, 'See the monster's gone and I'm here now.'

---

Mrs Linnet spends most of her waking hours listening to her radio. She 'hears' the voices of her dead husband and is generally happy with the 'conversations' she has with him. Occasionally though, the 'messages' upset or frighten her and she sits, melancholy and tearful. Staff of the hostel try to divert her attention by including her in the life of the unit, but she soon returns to listen intently to 'my husband'.

Appropriate medication might have decreased the intensity and frequency of Edward's hallucinations and those and Mrs Linnet.

## A world of confabulations

We discussed confabulating in Chapter 3. There are some people whose world is peppered with these imaginary stories. They are continually seeking explanations to fill in gaps in their memories. The people who confabulate are often the ones who enjoy 'chatting' and have a fund of stories to tell. To step into their world, you may have to do little more than listen and drop in an occasional question, but your interest will help the person feel important and add to their contentment.

> Mavis and Janet tell everyone that they have been coming to this 'guesthouse' since their children were small. (They have only known each other since they came to live in the recently built hostel a month or two ago.) They enjoy exchanging 'memories' about the outings they had and the people they met 'here' many years ago, and even recall different trees and furniture and architectural features, and weave stories around them. When they can find an interested listener, they are delighted.
>
> Often they are in their 'holiday' mood, and will ask staff to pack them a picnic lunch, so that they can revisit an old haunt. Then they eat it in the garden.
>
> Entering into the spirit of their confabulatory world helps greatly to keep these two women contented.

## In and out of the 'real' world

Sometimes we can be puzzled by the person who moves in and out of the real world; one minute delusional, confabulating or living in the past, and the next responding rationally to what is going on around or telling a story that is factual. Earlier we spoke of Evelyn (page 48) who confabulated just about all of the time. A very old lady, she would also tell stories that were outside the experience of younger staff but they were quite true. What made it harder for the listener to discriminate between imagination and fact was her distressed reaction if neither was believed.

Respond to everything as though it is real, but be aware that this is characteristic for that person.

# A distorted world

For some people, their worlds are completely distorted, with little or no contact with reality, persistently playing out no longer appropriate previous life-roles and habits, confused about location, sometimes 'living' in another town or country, at times in one building, at times in another, confabulating sometimes, delusional at others. They are often inappropriately practising bits of old skills and replacing people in their own lives with others around them. Mr Adams (Chapter 5) and Sister Edmond in the video 'Dementia with Dignity' lived in a totally distorted world.

> Sister Edmond believed that staff of the nursing home where she lived were her colleagues in some of the convents where she once lived, and that the nursing home was a convent. She confabulated, conducting a tour of the nursing home, explaining and describing how this room or that room used to be before they 'renovated' it. To her, the camera crew were people she once knew in the country town where she grew up as a child of a large family. She would talk to them about her brothers who 'you used to go fishing with', or sometimes jolly them along referring to them as her brothers. Sister Edmond talked of her mother and grandmother as though they were still alive and planned to visit them when she returned 'home'.
>
> She lived totally and contentedly in this distorted world. Sometimes there was a moment of bewilderment when her 'facts' did not seem to make sense, such as when there was some confusion about her brother's or her mother's age. This would quickly pass and she would happily continue her anecdotes.

When a person lives in this distorted world their underlying personality may not be greatly changed: an erstwhile dignified or an autocratic or a motherly person may still have those totally same personality traits. And while many are unaware of another reality besides their own, others give the impression that at times there is a grim and determined, but not quite conscious, struggle to hold on to 'normality'. By stepping into the person's distorted world, we can often ease that struggle.

---

**For people living in the strange, confused worlds of dementia, their world is the only reality.**

---

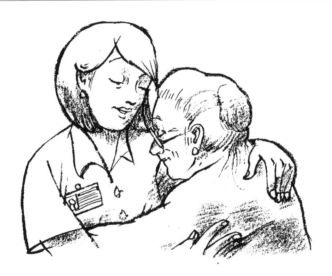

# MODELLING

---

A person with dementia may model themselves on you by copying your behaviour.

Attitudes and mannerisms are copied.

If the modelled behaviour is understanding and caring, relationships between staff and residents improve.

The person's self-esteem is enhanced by your approval of their behaviour.

---

# Using you as a model

A person with dementia observes the people around them and is often quick to pick up attitudes, mannerisms and behaviour. They often use another person as a model for their own behaviour. This can be turned to great advantage to expand the person's range of activity and social competence and promote better relationships with family, friends, staff and between residents.

When a person likes you and you approve of their behaviour, their confidence grows and they feel pleased with themself.

## *A copied attitude*

The three women who sit near the outside door are irritated by Bob, who no longer knows, and is beyond learning, how to manipulate handles and knobs. Several times a day he tries to go into the garden. Gripping the handle, he rattles the door. The women call to him to stop. 'Go away, go away', they tell him, as he becomes infuriated when the door fails to open.

For the next day or two the nurse quietly opens the door for him. 'There you are, Bob, you can go out now', each time turning to the women to say, 'He has forgotten how to open the door. He can't help it, you know.'

From then on, one or other of the women opens the door for Bob, explaining to anyone who cares to listen, 'He can't help it. He's forgotten.' Staff praise them for their caring attitude.

## *A copied behaviour*

Throughout her lifetime Gwen was a fashionable dresser. Since she came to the ward she has lost interest in herself, but she notices and comments when I wear a smart frock. I make sure that I visit her first thing in the morning and I seek her out each time I go to the ward. She stands back to admire my outfit and strokes my skirt, feeling the material between her fingers. Her approval comes in single words: 'Pretty', 'Nice'.

Gradually, she dresses with more care. I notice: 'Gwen, your blue dress is pretty', 'You have taken trouble to match your cardigan to your dress', or more often, 'You do look nice'.

A pleasant aside to this story is the humour Gwen perceives in our mutual admiration—as we exchange our compliments, she can hardly contain her laughter.

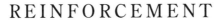

# REINFORCEMENT

**Preserve remaining memory and skills for as long as possible by reinforcing them with pleasant and repetitive experiences.**

**Reinforce with praise, repetition and the senses.**

**Praise emphasises approval of the person's actions. Praise promotes feelings of security by giving clear messages of what is acceptable.**

**Praise must be sincere and equal to the difficulty of what the person is trying to achieve.**

**Repetition reinforces identity, memories and behaviour.**

**Activities, outings, instructions, actions, gestures and finding the way around are more effective when repeated.**

**Emphasise words and actions by using the senses: sight, hearing, touch, smell, taste and rhythm.**

## Understanding reinforcement

The term 'reinforcement', both negative and positive, is used in a very special sense in connection with behaviour modification and reality therapy.

For our purpose, reinforcement means pleasant or repeated experiences which maintain the person's identity by strengthening remaining memory and skills, behaviour and social relationships for as long as possible. And, importantly, reinforcement lessens confusion and promotes the person's feelings of security and confidence by clearly indicating what is approved or not acceptable.

# Reinforce with praise

Praise puts the stamp of approval on the way a person acts. Praising spontaneous actions emphasises that it is all right to do that here.

Praise must be sincere. People affected by dementia can be perceptive about the sincerity of praise, becoming embarrassed and unbelieving if you overpraise, and aggrieved if you do not recognise their achievements.

Praise can range from a simple 'thank you', a smile and a nod of approval to publicly announcing the achievement and inviting applause from the group.

### Praise should equal the effort

The effort needed to undertake a task differs according to the person's remaining capacity and the difficulty of the task. The harder it is for the person to achieve what is being asked or what they are trying to do, the more the praise is earned.

The woman who controls her tears after trying for several weeks has put in more effort than, say, the man who likes to sweep the path each day. The sweeper will probably be bewildered by anything more than 'Thank you' or 'You did that well' each time he does the task, but the woman will proudly respond to extravagant praise the first time she gains control of her weeping.

### Decrease praise appropriately

Decrease the strength and amount of praise as the task or behaviour becomes more commonplace.

Let us look more closely at the tearful woman:

> Faith weeps every time she approaches or is greeted by a member of staff. Responding to her feelings of sadness, consoling her and diverting her attention do not have any impact. Staff, volunteers and family decide on a plan. Each time she cries we respond, 'No, Faith. I will go away while you're crying', or 'I'll come back to talk to you when you stop crying'. The first time she achieves this we make a fuss, praising and recognising how much effort it has cost her.

> We repeat but gradually decrease the praise, replacing words with a smile and a hug after about ten days, when it is commonplace for her not to cry.
>
> Faith's happier manner is the result of three pleasant experiences: first, our praise; second, the satisfaction she obtains from our continuing attention; and third, her increased acceptance into the social circle of other residents.
>
> She lapses on occasions, but a frown and an 'Uh-uh', prompt her to control herself.

## Reinforce by repetition

Repetition will strengthen a person's identity, memories and location, and enhance understanding. Repeat the person's name when addressing them, and repeat it to others at every appropriate opportunity. This reinforces self-identity and a sense of who they are to the people around.

### *Repeat activities*

Activities with repetitive components are more likely to be remembered and anticipated than those that change frequently. The person who knows it is her job to stir the ingredients has no apprehension about joining the cooking group. She has more chance of achieving a task she knows well and her self-esteem is enhanced.

A familiar bus trip, preferably to a park where there are a number of diversions—gardens, birds, animals and water—or walking frequently along the same route is likely to be remembered, talked about and looked forward to. Of course, this does not mean other excursions should not take place. Outings keep people in touch with the real world, are important and enjoyed, but the unfamiliar is less likely to be remembered.

Photographs and souvenirs prompt memories of outings and activities and reinforce the pleasure. Strong cardboard is a suitable base to which numbers of photographs can be attached. It can then be covered with plastic and placed on a wall for all to see. Flowers, leaves, postcards, admission tickets and other mementoes provide material for making scrapbooks and for reminiscing.

## Use the same words

It is not always possible to remember to use the same sentence, but the main word(s) of the message should be the same:

◆ 'bath', 'shower' or 'wash'
◆ 'lounge', 'TV room' or 'sitting room'
◆ 'pills' or 'tablets'
◆ 'medication' or 'medicine'

Instructions should be given with the same words. The actions and gestures of non-verbal communication should also be repeated often and consistently, so that they become familiar.

## Finding the way

The layout of the new location, such as a nursing home, is best taught by frequently going over the same route. 'Finding the way' is a necessary part of the familiarisation plan for every resident and should be consistently followed by all staff.

Start at a central point, say the dining room, and walk with the person. Take it slowly, bit by bit, stopping to emphasise the route where necessary.

'This is the dining room. Now we turn this way...see the picture of the children playing ball? Now walk along here past the kitchen, past the pink door...the green door...the white door...one, two, three doors. We go past the bathroom...See...the photographs on the wall...Here's your room...number 6... Here is the photograph of your son on the door, a blue door.'

Open the door, thus allowing them to recognise possessions. 'Here's your bedcover, oh, and the flowers your granddaughter brought you.' Allow time for the person's mind to absorb that this is their own room. Then return to the dining room, pointing out the same markers on the way.

Even though there is a lot to remember, with most people you will need to repeat this procedure for only a day or two.

## Reinforce by using the senses

Use the senses: seeing, hearing, touching, smelling, tasting and rhythm.

An example of a structured activity using sensation is flower arranging. The flowers are passed around, admired for colour and shape, touched for texture and smelled for perfume—sometimes even tasted when someone decides the roses look good enough to eat!

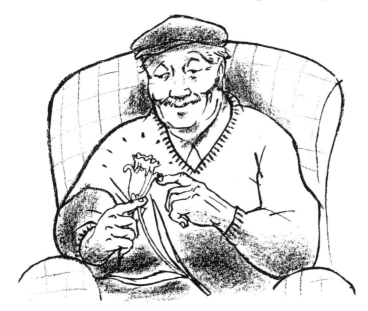

Selection of a vase requires seeing and touching, and discussing shape, surface, suitability and composition.

Using moment-to-moment opportunities is even more effective:

◆ 'It's spring! See the sunshine. Feel how warm it is on your face.'
◆ 'Mmmmmm—if you take a deep breath, you can smell spring in the air.'
◆ 'See the new leaves on the tree.'
◆ 'Taste the chocolate in the cake.'
◆ 'The coffee smells good.'

◆ 'Feel how soft your hands are.'

◆ 'The hand lotion smells nice...smell.'

Walks and outings provide many opportunities for experiencing sensations. There are so many sights and sounds, smells and textures and new food tastes.

A sense of rhythm is usually well preserved. Rhythm facilitates and reinforces movement by foot and finger tapping and body movement. Rhythmic movement strengthens awareness of where limbs and body are in space, particularly when dancing with a partner. A conga snake moving in rhythm is an effective activity to reinforce social closeness, body and limb movement and a sense of enjoyment.

### Use a dominant sense

Observe the person who uses one sense more than others; the one-time tailor who feels the texture of material between his fingertips, the erstwhile dressmaker who strokes the fall of a skirt, and the cook who 'tastes' the food. Make use of this dominant sense. Other examples are the woman who continually smells her cosmetics, the manicurist who likes to sort out nail-polish colours and the bookkeeper who reads and writes figures.

# HANDLING CHANGE

Change is unsettling and it often takes a long time to adjust to a new set of circumstances.

Even small changes can increase confusion for the dementing person already living in an uncertain world.

If change is introduced slowly, it is more likely to be accomplished effectively for all concerned.

Ideally a proposed change should be discussed and the person given a choice where possible. If the change involves a move, the person should be encouraged to help.

Find ways to make the change a pleasant experience.

A steady routine and good communication among staff minimises the need for frequent and unnecessary changes.

# Understanding the effects of change

Change is never easy. Change creates an inner turmoil, it is unsettling and it often takes us a long time to adjust to a new set of circumstances.

Remember how it was when you changed schools, or moved to a new town or a new country? Saying goodbye to old friends and familiar places is sad. You feel apprehensive and a little scared at the thought of facing a strange new experience. Will I like the teachers? Will the people in the new country accept me? Will I make friends? Will I get used to new surroundings? Will I adapt to new customs and rules?

## *Change adds to confusion*

At times we give too little consideration to the effects of change on the person with dementia, believing that they will not be sufficiently aware of the change for it to be meaningful. But imagine the effect of change on the dementing person already living in a world of uncertainties!

Even a simple change may worsen confusion: variations in your attitude; expectations that differ from one staff member to another; disapproval where someone else has approved; changes in key staff; morning activity moved for one day to the afternoon. Even changing the underwear drawer or rearranging furniture can cause bewilderment and distress.

> Jessie's husband moves her favourite chair across the sitting room to the window, and faces it away from the room with its familiar furnishings. Agitated, Jessie roams around the room, picking up things and putting them down. Then she leaves. Eventually she sits in the less comfortable chair in the place where her old chair used to be.

# Introduce change slowly

The dementing person may not be able to grasp the reason for change or comprehend why their comfortable life is being disarranged. To prevent a person from being overwhelmed by feelings of helplessness and anxiety, introduce change slowly and sensitively.

> Hettie went missing for two days and Joe knows it is now time for her to go to the nursing home. Each day he talks to her about leaving and reassures her that he will visit often. Hettie is distressed, but she understands. She helps pack the suitcases and selects a few personal possessions to take.
>
> When the nursing-home bed is available, Joe arranges the new room and spends some time each day with her until she feels less lost and forlorn.

# Handling change

> 'We've moved you to a nice single room. Come and have a look,' smiles the nurse when Mrs Perry returns from the bus trip.
>
> Shortly afterwards, Mrs Perry is discovered standing in the doorway of the new room with one of her still packed suitcases, whimpering 'Go home, go home'. Usually a gentle, cooperative woman, she cannot be comforted. Reluctant to go to bed she is found in the early hours of the morning wandering on another floor of the nursing home.
>
> 'I'm disappointed. I thought you would be grateful. I went to a lot of trouble to get this room for you,' grumbles the nurse. She moves Mrs Perry back to the old room, which she has shared with two other women since moving to the hostel six months ago.

Let us examine how Mrs Perry's room change might be accomplished more successfully.

### *Giving a choice*

Allow Mrs Perry to have some control; give her a choice. Is the change essential? She may not wish to leave her room companions.

### *Getting her used to the idea*

As soon as the proposed change is decided upon, gently but repeatedly discuss it with Mrs Perry, and also with the other residents so that they too become used to the idea. Encourage relatives to talk with her about the move. Allow the new room to remain vacant for as long as possible so that she has the opportunity to become familiar with it. This may take only one day.

If she is anxious, try to find the specific reason and deal with it. Maybe a simpler, clearer explanation may be necessary.

### Ask her to help

Do not make the move in her absence. Coming home to find her familiar private world has changed is likely to precipitate a catastrophic reaction. Invite a family member to help. Encourage her to help with the packing. She may not contribute much, but she will feel useful and important.

Make the move a pleasant, chatty experience.

### Settling in

Do not leave her surrounded by packed suitcases and boxes. If you are needed elsewhere and there is no one else to help, suggest you both come back later to unpack.

To accelerate her adjustment to the new room, place belongings and store clothing in positions as close as possible to the previous ones. If the layout of the room is significantly different, help her to familiarise herself. It may take a few days. If it is necessary, accompany her to the dining room and other facilities until she is used to the changed direction. Watch for signs of anxiety.

Taken gently and with support from staff, residents and family, change can be fairly smooth.

# An unavoidable change

When an unplanned change cannot be avoided, such as admission to hospital, follow as many of these guidelines as you can. In particular, discuss the change. The person may understand more than you think.

You are leaving a unit where you have been working for twelve months? Talk about it with the residents so that they become accustomed to the idea. The dining room and craft room are to be interchanged? Tell the residents. They might like to help with the move.

## *Going to hospital*

For all of us, there are times when hospitalisation for surgery or other procedures is essential. Hospital staff seldom have the time necessary to deal with the anxiety and sometimes abject fear of the person with dementia, or to contain the frequent crying and calling out to other patients.

In addition, the relationship between hospital staff and the person with dementia is often strained because of the way the person acts and the staff members' lack of experience in dealing with the effects of dementia.

Where possible, the prospective patient should be accompanied to, and settled into, the hospital by a person who is familiar to them and who knows how they will react, preferably a family member. Most hospitals appreciate the presence of such a person visiting as often and for as long as possible.

---

**A steady routine and continued communication among staff minimise the need for frequent and unnecessary change.**

---

CHAPTER NINE

# Caring

In this edition I have addressed the 'Caring at home' section of this chapter to the family or home caregiver, while the sections 'Moving into a nursing home or hostel' and 'Settling in' are also in part addressed to professional care workers. However, both sections are equally applicable to carer and care worker. The remainder of this chapter, while mainly for professional care workers, will also be of interest to the home carer.

## AT HOME

The home carer needs maximum assistance and emotional support from family, friends and community services.

The more rest and recreation the carer obtains, the longer it is possible for the dementing person to stay at home. Day care, respite care and family and friends allow the primary carer to have time out.

Help in the home is available from home nursing services, Home Care, Meals on Wheels and community and neighbourhood centres. Contact the area Aged Care Assessment Team (ACAT) for suggestions about the services available in the local district.

Advice about equipment and aids is available from physiotherapy and occupational therapy departments and organisations such as Independent Living Centres.

A social worker will act as a reference point for financial, legal and community care, as well as offering trained counselling. Alzheimer's Associations and the Carers' Association offer group support.

Some nursing homes and dementia hostels encourage relatives to form support groups.

# Caring for the home carer

In the advanced stages of the illness the home carer is looking after a person whose confusion and memory loss are severe and whose behaviour is at best strange and unfamiliar and at worst disruptive and difficult to handle.

In order to cope the carer at home will require as much assistance and emotional support as possible from family, friends and community services. Planning six or twelve months ahead and establishing a network of supports helps the carer to organise her or his life and goes some way to relieving the stress of caring.

To ease the strain a little, the carer will benefit from regular breaks and a holiday or a long time out at least once a year. There are a number of services that the home carer can call on to help with the caring of the person with dementia and these are discussed later in this chapter.

# Caring for the person with dementia

In previous chapters we have explored a number of suggestions for handling the behaviour and symptoms of the person with dementia. Here are other suggestions to handle situations that face the home carer.

# Telling the person of the diagnosis

'How do I handle telling her?' 'What do I say if he is upset?'

To tell or not to tell is a dilemma for many families.

It is probably best to be guided by the way the person has dealt with adversity in the past. Someone who has always coped well with life's obstacles will probably be easier to tell than someone who has always been overwhelmed by trouble.

You will also need to consider that:

◆ A person with a life-threatening condition does have the right to know so that they can have some control over the decisions being made about their future. It also gives them the opportunity to order their affairs, such as making a will and negotiating an enduring power of attorney and enduring guardianship, while still able to do so.

◆ The person will know that something is wrong and not being able to talk about it will only increase anxiety, which may lead to depression or symptoms of stress.

If the carer or other family member cannot bring themself to talk to the affected person about the diagnosis, ask the family doctor, specialist or other professional to do so.

# Incontinence

Incontinence is a major problem for the home carer and it worsens as the disease progresses. Incontinence can be due to a number of reasons and should be properly assessed by a doctor or gerontological nurse.

### Infection

Consult the family doctor when loss of bladder control occurs in order to determine whether there is a urinary tract infection. Appropriate treatment may cure the condition.

### Other factors

Emotional distress can also be a reason for loss of control. When the dementing person is upset about something in their day-to-day life, incontinence may increase.

Incontinence may also be due to slowness of movement (the person is unable to reach the toilet in time), physical incapacity or a short time span between the brain signalling the need to go and the release of urine.

Someone who is disoriented may be unable to find the bathroom, in particular when they are confused after waking at night. A night-light and a commode chair beside the bed or, if the toilet is close by, a handrail from bed to toilet are useful.

Difficulty with zips, buttons and pants often results in accidents. Velcro fastenings are easier to manage.

### Preventive toileting

It is better not to give a drink in the two hours before bedtime. Two-or three-hour toileting helps, but it is not always effective because not everyone urinates to the same time pattern. To obtain a personal pattern, make a note of the liquid drunk and the times of urination over a period of about two weeks.

Time the visit to the toilet ten minutes before the estimated time that the person will urinate and they will usually oblige and accidents will decrease.

When soiling is a problem, first consult a medical practitioner to establish whether there is a physical cause. Sometimes the person's bowel movement is fairly regular and taking them to the toilet beforehand may save mishaps.

### Clothing and appliances

Tracksuits, back-divided dresses and slips, and drip-dry garments are suggested to cut down on laundry when there is frequent wetting or soiling.

A range of absorbent pants, pads and bed sheets is readily available. However, appliances such as bags, tubing and catheters are seldom successful for the dementing person. Some people strenuously resist having the appliance fitted, or tear it off once it is in place.

A number of pamphlets and booklets dealing with incontinence are available. Enquire at your local Community Health Centre.

# Walking exercise

Exercise is important for physical health, inducing sleep and satisfying the person's desire to walk.

Some dementing people have an excellent sense of location and should be encouraged to continue with routine walking. Accompanying the walker for a stroll around the streets or in the park will ease apprehension about the risk of the person wandering away.

## The pacer and wanderer

Some people who wander are quite content to wander around the house until they tire. Others will pace restlessly looking for means of 'escape'. Restricting or restraining someone who has an urge to walk often results in frustration, aggression and sometimes violence. The person who repeatedly tries to go outside often rattles locks, strikes their fists against the door and even turns their wrath on the carer.

Where there is a large backyard, with secure fences and high gates on each side, it will often be sufficient space to satisfy the incessant walker and may decrease the urge for someone to wander away. Sometimes even a secure path at the side of the house will satisfy them temporarily. Of course not everybody has an outside space and the inside space may not be suitable for walking.

Taking the person for a walk is the only solution. Respite care workers are sometimes available on an hourly basis for walking exercise. Contact your local ACAT for information.

## Identification

It is a worry for the home carer that someone might suddenly take it into their head to wander away: this is always a possibility. When the person is at risk of wandering away and becoming lost, attach a permanent wrist bracelet. There are several different types available. Name, address and telephone number should be clearly marked. A name and address card in a protective cover in the top pocket or in a handbag is also likely to be found. Attaching a label to the person's back is not necessary or desirable as it may well make them a spectacle and a figure of fun.

Have a photograph and description of the dementing person readily available in case the police need to be notified. This allows for quick identification when someone is found wandering far from home.

There are some devices that are said to be effective in tracking a person who is lost. Enquire from your local ACAT or Alzheimer's Association.

# Mobility problems

Where the carer experiences difficulty managing the person with a physical problem, such as slow or painful movement, unsteadiness, falling or immobility, a correct medical diagnosis and appropriate treatment of the problem is essential. Occupational therapists and physiotherapists will advise on aids and equipment and physical treatment when the medical diagnosis is confirmed.

## *Equipment*

To assist the person with a physical disability a range of special equipment and aids is available. Wheelchairs, commodes, orthopaedic chairs, quad sticks and other equipment can be hired from some hospital physiotherapy and occupational therapy departments and private suppliers.

Advice about design, manufacture and installation of special equipment can also be obtained from these professionals and organisations such as Independent Living Centres.

Financial help to hire or purchase equipment and aids, where needed, is available in some circumstances. Hospital social work departments and community centres will provide information.

## *Handrails*

Rails installed beside steps, bath, toilet and in the shower recess provide support and enhance the person's feeling of security.

A portable frame that fits around the toilet makes it easier for the person to sit and stand, as do elevated seats that fit firmly on top of the toilet bowl.

## *Chairs*

A recliner chair is handy. Sleep can often be induced more readily in this sort of chair than in a bed. Reclining also provides a change of position when the person spends much of the time sitting.

Orthopaedic chairs with adjustable legs and rigid arms facilitate standing and sitting, and some can be fitted with a tray for meals.

Some cane and wicker chairs are comfortable, but it is necessary to protect frail skin from injury by fitting a protective covering, preferably padded, over the armrests.

### Shower

A flexible hose shower and a special chair where the person can sit while showering is necessary where there are problems with balance, standing and movement. Removing the step at the shower entrance lessens the risk of falling and access for wheelchairs is made easier if shower-recess doors are removed.

# Aids

A range of aids is available for walking, eating, gardening and other activities.

### Walking aids

Walking sticks, frames and quad sticks will support the person who finds it difficult to walk. Before contemplating the purchase of a walking aid, however, make sure the person can use it. Often the dementing person has reached a stage where they have lost the ability to co-ordinate the required movements, for example the lifting and placing of a walking frame.

### Eating aids

Specially designed cutlery, rimmed plates and bowls that reduce the risk of spilling, non-slip suction pads and special drinking aids can be purchased at pharmacies and specialty departments.

# Home care

It will be of great benefit to the home caregiver if they establish a network of supports as early as possible in the course of the dementia.

## *Family support*

In some families there is considerable support for the home carer with relatives taking a turn looking after the person in order to give the carer a much-needed break. Where family members are disinclined at first to take part in the caring it is probably because they have not understood the true nature of dementia. In such instances, often a group session or consultation with a professional helps to develop some understanding and people are then agreeable to lend support for the caregiver. Hospital social work departments, psychologists and Alzheimer's and Carers' Associations can usually provide this service.

## *Home nursing*

Community nursing services will assess the type of nursing help required. The nurse will administer injections, apply dressings, and supervise a medication regimen and attend to special bath and hygiene requirements. As a regular visitor, the nurse is in a position to pick up health and management problems at an early stage. Contact nursing services direct or through the Community Health Centre in your district, ACAT or doctor.

Other health services such as physiotherapy, occupational therapy and podiatry are also available to help the person with dementia to stay independent.

## *Help in the home*

The Commonwealth Government in partnership with State governments provides a range of services through Home and Community Care (HACC) and other service organisations. Fees for these services are calculated on a means-test basis. There are also a number of private agencies that offer a variety of services, for which the user pays the full cost of the service, and community aid agencies which provide help free of charge or for a minimal fee. Services vary from one locality to another and include house cleaning, gardening, lawnmowing, household repairs, shopping, person-sitting and home modification. Community aid and neighbourhood centres may offer transport, person-sitting, shopping or other services that might not be provided by government-funded or private agencies.

Information about the types of home help offered is available at Home Care Centres, Community Health Centres, ACATs and hospital social work departments. The caregiver should always check as to what assistance they are entitled to, for example, from the Veterans' Affairs Department in the case of a returned serviceman or war widow.

### *Meals*

Where the carer is having difficulty or the person with dementia is living alone, a meal can be delivered five days a week by Meals on Wheels. Meals are provided by local councils, hospitals or community groups, depending on where the person lives. Some cultural and religious organisations cater for special dietary needs. A charge is usually levied for home-delivered meals.

## Rest for the carer

Caring for the person in the advanced stages of dementia is physically and emotionally draining. It is important for all caregivers to establish a network of people and services to assist them so that they obtain sufficient rest and recreation. Otherwise they may become exhausted and be at risk of physical and emotional breakdown.

One way of ensuring that the home carer looks after themself is to make a plan at least six months ahead.

◆ Allow for time out each week to go to the cinema or shopping, visit a friend or catch up on some sleep. Or just find a quiet corner to read a book. You might even gain some satisfaction in catching up with a household chore that you haven't had the time or energy to do. Plan specific activities ahead.

◆ Plan a holiday each year while the person with dementia is booked into a nursing home or hostel for respite care. You might like to just stay home and enjoy the peace and quiet of the house and garden. Be firm with yourself. Do not visit the respite facility each day!

◆ Write your plan on to a sheet of paper and place it where it is visible.

◆ So that you discipline yourself to follow your plan, make a contract with yourself that every time you do not keep to an item you will pay a forfeit. One man I know gave $10 (which he could ill afford) to St Vincent de Paul as his forfeit!

## Sleep

Often overlooked is the carer's lack of sleep. Carers may sleep fitfully, often half-awake listening for the sound of the person they are caring for. Where partners sleep in the same bed it is even harder for the 'well' partner to have a restful night's sleep; incontinence often requiring a change of clothes and bed linen once or twice during the night. Then there is the person who sleeps during the day and is awake all night. Under these circumstances the partner may be seriously deprived of sleep, caring for the person all night and having to snatch bits of sleep in between the daily demands on their time.

It is essential that the carer obtain sufficient rest. In some districts agencies offer night respite care either in the person's own home or in a residential facility. Family members will at times give a night to care for their relative; by sharing this task around the family they may only need to give one night every so often.

## Time out

It is beneficial and even necessary for the caregiver to have regular 'time out' to pursue their own interests. As we discussed earlier, to gain the most advantage from the break, it is important to plan how to spend the time. In order that the time away is untroubled by the urge to rush home, ensure that the sitter is familiar with the dementing person's needs and is prepared for and able to handle emotional outbursts or other crises.

## Help from family and friends

See also above: *Rest for the carer*. The carer may be reluctant to impose on others but more often than not family members or close friends are willing to share the caring. A round table discussion or group consultation with a professional will often result in a satisfactory arrangement.

Some family members and friends roster themselves regularly for a few hours while others come when they are able. The pressure on the carer is alleviated, thus enabling the dementing person to remain at home for a longer period. Respite carers can also be employed from reputable private agencies or sometimes through community agencies.

Not far from where I live an elderly lady did a letterbox drop for a few streets around about her house, appealing for an hour a month's support from neighbours. She gained enough hours' help to enable her husband to be cared for at home until his death.

## Day respite care

In some districts, day respite is provided in special dementia day centres from one to five days a week. Day centres for elderly people with no cognitive impairment will sometimes accept a dementing person if there is no risk of him or her wandering away or behaving in a disruptive manner. Some set aside a day or two days a week to cater for people with dementia.

Nursing homes and dementia care hostels on occasions have a day centre attached. The benefit of these centres is that when one of their members is accepted into residential care there, both the person and the carer is already familiar with the facility.

Diversional therapists or recreational workers are often employed by day centres and a range of activities and outings is undertaken. The centre may ask for a small donation; some are free while others make a small charge to cover the cost of meals.

Many centres have their own buses or volunteer drivers, but on occasions transport has to be arranged by the home carer.

## Respite accommodation

The person with dementia can be accepted for respite care in a hostel or nursing home for up to sixty-three days in any one financial year, allowing the carer to have a holiday or a break at home for a well-earned rest. This can be extended by twenty-one days if necessary. Because of the heavy demand on respite beds, it is advisable to book ahead. Respite care to meet emergencies can usually be found.

In most instances respite accommodation is in a regular nursing home or dementia hostel. However, there are facilities in some States especially established to cater only for respite care, including people with dementia.

# Emotional support for the carer

Carers are often emotionally stressed and invariably have mixed feelings about the illness and the dementing person. At times they may become frustrated, angry and depressed, or even fearful of contracting the disease. There may be no family member to call on or no one prepared to help. Sometimes the dementia of a parent is a trigger for or exacerbation of family conflict and this places extra pressure on the home carer.

Many carers feel too proud to seek help or feel that by doing so they are admitting to failure. Once over the first hurdle of seeking help, they will usually find great comfort in their contact with a support group or a professional counsellor.

## *Professional consultation*

There are a number of professionals who specialise in assisting the carer. Counsellors with various training backgrounds and specialising in dementia care are now employed throughout Australia and are attached to Aged Care Assessment Teams, and some community centres and carers' associations such as the Alzheimer's Association and Carers' Association. Some of these services are government funded and are offered free of charge; some practise privately and charge a recommended fee. It is advisable that the carer be assured of the appropriate training of the counsellor they are being referred to.

Doctors who are regularly seeing the person with dementia and the carer will sometimes be the appropriate person to help through periods of emotional stress. A psychiatric or psychological consultation may be indicated.

## *The social worker*

Linking the carer with a social worker at the earliest possible time provides ongoing counselling and emotional support in times of crisis. The social worker will also act as a reference point for practical, financial and legal help, home help and day and respite care options.

### Alzheimer's Associations

Alzheimer's Associations under various names are part of a world-wide organisation providing support for families and friends of persons with dementia. Support groups meet regularly in city and country locations to give mutual support, learn about the illness and share experiences.

### The Carers' Association

The Carers' Association is a nationwide organisation with branches in all states and territories which offers support to any carer regardless of the handicap or illness of the person being cared for. Some of these groups meet within nursing homes.

### Other groups

Some community agencies and social work departments in nursing homes and hospitals conduct groups, which home carers are welcome to attend. Some residential facilities encourage relatives to form support groups, which at times have close contact and act in an advisory capacity to the administration of the unit.

## Financial and legal matters

Matters of finance and legal affairs are of utmost importance when someone is affected by dementia. Organisations such as the Alzheimer's Association and the Carers' Association can advise as to the appropriate department or professional to consult for specialised financial advice. Where business affairs are concerned it is imperative that a solicitor be consulted as early as possible in the course of the illness. The negotiation of an enduring power of attorney is of utmost importance for the wellbeing and protection of both the person with dementia and the family.

In general matters of finance, Centrelink offers a free Financial

Information Service to help carers improve their standard of living by using their money to its best advantage. People eligible for this service are those who are receiving or about to apply for a Social Security Pension, receiving a Veterans' Affairs Pension or those who are planning to retire.

# Financial matters

## *Carer Pension*

The carer who is providing full-time care for the person with dementia should contact Centrelink in their area to determine their eligibility for a Carer Pension and other benefits. A carer who is already in receipt of an Aged Pension or other pension will not be entitled to receive this pension.

Someone who is not otherwise entitled to pension benefits may be eligible for a special benefit. A Pensioner Concession Card entitles the holder to a range of health benefits. As well as health benefits, a Veterans' Affairs Gold Card entitles the person to a wide range of services free of charge.

If the carer has any difficulty with pension payments contact Centrelink, either at the local office or directly to the State office or seek advice from one of the carers' associations or a professional consultant.

## *Domiciliary Nursing Care Benefit*

This is a benefit paid by the Commonwealth Department of Health and Family Services. It is not means-tested and is paid to, amongst others, carers of people with severe dementia who require full-time nursing care at home. Application forms for this benefit are available from a community nurse, doctor, Community Health Centre, and State or Territory branches of the Department of Health and Family Services.

## *Bank accounts*

Informal arrangements can usually be made by a spouse or next of kin with the bank to draw on the person's account. However it is preferable to have the dementing person's authority if they are competent to sign this. If the carer has an enduring power of attorney, this should be presented to the bank as the authority to operate the account. If the account is in joint names with an authority for both to withdraw, the carer will not need another document.

# Legal matters

Matters such as making a will, assigning an enduring power of attorney and sorting out business and other financial matters should be negotiated while the person with dementia has the legal competence to do so.

## *Competence*

Where someone is considered to be incompetent such as in the case of the person with dementia, matters such as making a will, making decisions about treatment, finances and business affairs are of utmost importance.

A person with dementia may be sufficiently competent to make some decisions, such as indicating their wishes in a will, but quite unable to sort out the implications of surgery of a serious nature. Where there is a need for a decision of some complexity or where legal or major financial matters are concerned, it is important that the person's competence to make that particular decision is determined.

The assessment of a person's competence should always be done by a trained and experienced person.

## *Enduring power of attorney*

If the dementing person owns property, investments or deposits of money, either alone or jointly with the spouse, or if they are engaged in any business arrangement, the carer should immediately see a solicitor for advice on obtaining an enduring power of attorney. A power of attorney can only be delegated by a person who fully understands its significance and it should be negotiated as early as possible in the illness.

Failing all else, the Protective Office or similar legal authority will undertake to manage the financial affairs of a protected person. This protection is often conducted in association with the family, solicitor, business partner or other interested person.

The family carer should contact the Protective Office, a family solicitor, social worker, a carers' organisation, Community Legal Centre or Clerk of the Local Court for advice regarding the procedure for protection.

## *Guardianship*

Where there is no one responsible, or the person with dementia objects to proposed treatment that is necessary for their wellbeing, a guardian may be appointed by the Guardianship Tribunal.* This guardian may be the family carer. Such a carer can make this application directly to the Office of the Public Guardian, the Guardianship Tribunal or it can be conducted through a solicitor, community organisation or a professional person.

Where a guardian is appointed, that person has the responsibility for decisions regarding appropriate accommodation and medical and dental treatment where the person does not have the capacity to consent.

A recent change to the *Guardianship Act* in New South Wales now allows for people who want to plan ahead and who wish to have future control over their own lives to appoint an enduring guardian themselves. They can give the person they appoint as many responsibilities to act for them as they wish or they can appoint more than one enduring guardian. For instance, a man may wish to appoint his wife to look after all domestic arrangements and his solicitor or accountant to supervise his business interests. However, the authority to override the person's objections to medical treatment is a decision that can only be made by the Guardianship Tribunal. Contact the Office of the Public Guardian or equivalent in your State for further information.

---

*The Guardianship Tribunal in New South Wales determines if a person with a disability is incapable of making his or her own decisions and has need of a guardian. The tribunal also decides who the guardian should be. The Public Guardian is the guardian of last resort and when appointed by the tribunal is given authority to make certain lifestyle decisions for the person.

# MOVING TO A NURSING HOME OR HOSTEL

The carer and family may need assistance to make an informed decision.

Counselling is often helpful.

Involve the person with dementia in the planning where possible.

Offer a choice of units for the family to assess and place the person's name on a waiting list.

Prepare for the move gradually with occasional discussions and familiarisation with the chosen unit. Encourage the dementing person to help with the packing.

If the person refuses to go and all attempts at persuasion fail, applying for guardianship may be the only way to transfer them.

The person being moved from hospital to a unit should be prepared for the transfer.

Have a functional assessment and personal profile or similar assessments completed and take or send them with other records to the nursing home or hostel.

## Making the decision

As the illness progresses, caring for the person at home may become too difficult. Incontinence, confusion, wandering away and disruptive or other behaviour makes life difficult, especially when the person no longer recognises the carer or their home surroundings. The whole situation may become unmanageable. As well, the caregiver may be simply too tired to continue. There may be a crisis. The home carer may now be forced to consider nursing home or hostel accommodation.

It is advisable for the home carer not to rush into deciding about residential care, if possible. Discussing it with a trained person will give an overview of the available options for residential care and an opportunity to discuss their feelings about the proposed move.

## How the carer feels

I have never known a carer who has not had mixed feelings about making the decision to move the dementing person to a nursing home or hostel. They may feel unable to carry on but argue with themselves that they might be able to try a little harder. They are distressed if the relative no longer recognises them. They hope the person will improve and are encouraged by the occasional 'good' days or flashes of logic and memory.

They feel guilty. Didn't their marriage vows say 'in sickness and in health'? Isn't it wrong to 'put someone away'? Will people accuse them of 'dumping' their relative?

## Cultural attitudes

Some cultures have strong attitudes towards institutional care. Conflicts surface where, say, the cultural expectation is that a daughter will devote her life to caring for her father or mother in times of need. On the other hand, the daughter might favour residential care so that she can live an independent life like the women in her adopted country. Or she may have a young family who are her priority for care.

The appropriate ethnic agency will give advice where there is such a problem.

## Counselling the carer

Before the practicalities of accommodation can be attended to, the home carer will probably benefit from talking to someone who understands how they feel and who can help sort out their emotions. A referral to a social worker or counsellor who specialises in dementia with whom they may be able to talk freely, or to their general practitioner or psychiatrist, will help. Alzheimer's Association groups offer the support of others who have been through a similar experience. It often takes several discussions to reduce the intensity of the carer's feelings so that they are in the frame of mind to make a decision.

Counselling should continue to be available and accessible, at least until the carer becomes used to the person's new environment.

## Family involvement

While some families or individual members give unconditional support to the caregiver, others may not agree with the notion of the nursing home or hostel accommodation. They may not even appreciate the true nature of the illness or the weight of the burden of caring.

A meeting with the whole family informs members about both the illness and options for residential care. It gives them an opportunity to air their feelings and sort out differences of opinion and provides a climate of support for each member.

## Including the person with dementia

People have a right to know and to have some control over what is happening to them. Even though someone may only vaguely comprehend, it is better for them to be involved.

Where the person with dementia has known of their diagnosis and if they have been given the opportunity early in the course of the dementia to express their wishes about future care, they may have become used to the idea of nursing home accommodation. Including the dementing person in the discussion and decision making from the earliest possible moment may cut down on the trauma when the time comes for them to transfer to the facility.

## Emotional reaction

An emotional reaction is normal and to be expected. The person must be allowed to express these feelings and reassurance from the caregiver will ease the stress of the proposed separation. Mentioning the move occasionally and understanding from the carer will help them become used to the idea. Negative reactions will lessen and transition from home to unit is likely to be easier.

> Mr Grace's family occasionally discusses the move to a dementia unit and explains that 'Mum' can no longer look after him. At the day centre he tells them: 'I'm finished. I'm finished now.' At home he tries to give away his clothes and personal possessions. He refuses to speak to his wife.

> The family and the day-centre staff recognise that he feels abandoned and depressed. They encourage him to air his feelings and reassure him of their support. **,**

## Choosing the unit

If the need for residential care is not urgent, the home carer should take time in choosing the unit to suit the needs of the person with dementia and the family. With nursing-home fees now the responsibility of the person themself and their family, and large entrance fees being asked, the carer should use their discretion when choosing a residential facility for their relative. The practice of hospital nursing staff choosing a hostel or nursing home and shipping the patient off without reference to the carer or the person themself should now be past.

In situations where an urgent nursing home space is needed and the carer is not satisfied, a transfer can be arranged when a more suitable place becomes vacant. The lump-sum fee is transferable.

A special-purpose dementia hostel is better suited to the person who is mobile. Until an adequate number of hostels is built, however, some active people still have to be accommodated in nursing homes.

### *Assessing the unit*

In order to choose a unit, the family should visit two or three of those recommended as suitable. They should observe the following:

◆ Is it bright, comfortable, clean and free from unpleasant or strong disinfectant odours?
◆ Is the atmosphere relaxed?
◆ How do staff relate to residents and vice versa?
◆ Are the residents interested, chatting and occupied? Do they appear to be sedated, regimented? Are they tied into chairs?
◆ Do you feel welcome?
◆ Is the unit located a reasonable distance from home? Is there convenient public transport?

Once the family is satisfied that the unit is a possibility, they should find out:

- Exactly how much is charged?
- What are the extra charges?
- Are there outings and activities? And if so, what sort?
- Is a recreation worker or occupational or diversional therapist employed?
- What are the rules about visiting, taking out the resident or having an occasional meal with them?
- What clothing, possessions and furniture are allowed?
- What are the laundry arrangements?
- Does the unit welcome input from relatives? Can they assist as volunteers? Is there a relatives group?

The carer should not be backward about asking questions to make sure that the facility is suitable to their needs. If there is not an immediate vacancy, the person's name should be placed on the waiting list of one or more units of the family's choice. Some units accept residents in strict order of application and others on assessment of need. Most will give priority in emergency situations.

# Preparation to move

Like all changes, preparation to move to a residential facility should be gradual. Talk about it from time to time. It is better, however, not to emphasise it to the point where greater anxiety is caused. Mention it casually. The person will respond if he or she wants to talk about it.

### *Becoming familiar with the unit*

When someone is able to attend a day centre attached to a dementia unit, he or she becomes accustomed to the staff and residents and is familiar with the routine. Transition from home to unit then is fairly smooth. Unfortunately there are too few day centres attached to nursing homes and hostels, and not all will accept a resident just because they have attended the day centre.

Some nursing homes and hostels have a familiarisation procedure. The prospective resident is invited to attend regularly for a few hours, join in activities and stay for the midday meal. The transfer is then gradual and not so difficult for the person, family and staff. Even the occasional visit before the move can assist adjustment.

## *Packing*

Encourage the person to help with packing and the selection of clothes, possessions and photographs. Favourite belongings should be included: an old coat, a wallet, a bunch of old keys, a handbag, music-case or briefcase.

*Include money.* Handling money has special significance. Most people gain a feeling of satisfaction from having a few coins in a purse or wallet or the sound of money clinking in the pocket. Self-esteem also benefits from the independence of being able to phone home at will and pay for small purchases. Even when money or its value is not recognised, its use is often understood. Remember the woman in Chapter 5 who 'tips' the staff with old lottery tickets provided by her husband.

# Refusal to go

The person with dementia may have forgotten earlier discussions about the move to a residential facility. There may be a crisis and the family has not had time to prepare her or him. They feel frightened and abandoned. They refuse to go.

## *Persuasion*

Some families find it easier to tell the person they are going for a holiday or into hospital for treatment. While this sort of explanation may be the only way to get the person there, be prepared for them to take a long time to settle into new surroundings and staff have to deal with the person's distress. Catastrophic reactions in these circumstances are common. Eventually, the person will have to be told that he or she is not returning home.

## *Other measures*

Occasionally, and despite the most sensitive handling, someone determinedly refuses to leave and may physically resist all attempts to take them from home. The doctor, social worker or visiting health worker may be able to convince them. If this fails, the Guardianship Tribunal (see previous section) or similar legal authority may have to be involved to negotiate the transfer.

### *Medication is not desirable*

Administering heavy drug dosages so that the dementing person is not conscious of the move creates serious problems when the person wakes, frightened, in a strange place.

# Transferring from hospital

Sometimes the first indication that someone is dementing is when they are admitted to hospital with conditions associated with malnutrition or an injury. A social assessment confirms the person's inability to live alone and a move to a nursing home or dementia hostel is suggested to the family.

The hospitalised person needs preparation for the move similar to that of the person transferring from home.

### *A very unsatisfactory transfer*

> Shouting and struggling, hitting out with two plastic bags of belongings, Mr Fear resists the ambulance bearer's attempts to assist him through the front door of the nursing home.
>
> Nobody can persuade him to enter. He sits on the step in the rain alternately demanding 'What place is this?' and insisting he be taken home.
>
> Several hours pass before his family arrives to coax him to 'stay one night'.

*Mistake* The hospital staff do not include Mr Fear in the discussion with his family about transferring him to a nursing home: 'His brain's gone, he won't understand.'

*Mistake* The family is told not to bother accompanying him: 'He won't know the difference.'

*Mistake* When he is delivered to the ambulance, Mr Fear is told he is going home.

*Later mistake* His family tells him they will take him home in the morning.

## *His reactions*

Arriving at a strange place, Mr Fear is terrified and has a catastrophic reaction. When his family finally coax him inside the unit, they promise to take him home in the morning. He remembers this and persistently demands to go. His anxiety level is high and he is depressed for a long while. It is a long and difficult time before he settles in to the unit.

## *Staff reaction*

Staff members are angry and upset. They blame both the hospital staff and the family for Mr Fear's distress and take some time to develop a relationship with the relatives.

# Documents

To enable unit staff to provide the person with the best possible care and consideration, send or take all appropriate documents and reports. There may be a reason, for example if the person moves to a unit some distance from home, for them or his family to need to choose another doctor. Medical reports should be forwarded to the new doctor either before the person moves or as soon as possible after transfer.

## *Functional assessment*

An assessment of the person's functioning indicates what the person is capable of doing and what they do in fact do. It gives an idea, for example, how they manage to bath, dress, eat, walk, sit and so on, and how well they carry out these tasks. An assessment will also evaluate personality, behaviour and intellectual ability. Most dementia assessment and diagnostic clinics use specially designed functional assessments and a number of standard formats are available.

The functional assessment is best prepared by an occupational therapist or visiting nurse while the person still lives at home.

## *Personal profile* *

The personal profile tells us about the person, rather than what he or she can do. It is not a social history and the information is not confidential. The personal profile is available to all members of staff.

It should be compiled by a social worker from the Aged Care Assessment Team or dementia clinic or a health worker known to the family. Alternatively, the unit may prefer that the profile be completed by its own social worker or another appropriate staff member.

# Pension

In some situations, the dementing person is entitled to a single rate pension when they transfer to a nursing home or hostel. Apply to Centrelink or consult a social worker as soon as the person moves in.

# SETTLING IN †

It takes time for someone to settle in to new and unfamiliar surroundings. This can be from one week to several weeks.

If the transfer from home to unit is steady, it is more likely to be accomplished with a minimum of fuss.

On the first day, time spent with the new resident and relative will relieve some of their stress.

If the relative stays until the resident is asleep, the day will be easier for everyone.

The new resident who is alone needs extra attention from the staff to help with settling.

The person is settling when they attempt to find their way around, join in the life of the unit and make friends, and begin to trust staff.

---

* See Appendix A.
† Refer also to the section 'Handling change' in Chapter 8.

> **Expect an emotional reaction from the new resident. This is part of the settling-in process.**
>
> **The person with no immediate memory or one who has not been prepared for the move is more likely to become depressed or have a severe emotional reaction.**
>
> **Make families welcome. Discuss concerns as they arise.**

If the moving and settling in to the unit are accomplished steadily the transfer from home to a nursing home or a dementia hostel will be accomplished with a minimum of fuss and will be more satisfactory for the new resident, family and staff.

Moving from home to a residential facility is a major change in a person's life. Often too little consideration is given to the impact of such a move on the person with dementia. It is often assumed that they are not sufficiently aware for the move to have an effect. But how much more traumatic must it be for someone who may not fully comprehend what is happening to them?

# On arrival

## *Welcome*

Staff should devote some private uninterrupted time to the newly arrived person and relative. Welcome them to the facility.

If they have not had a preliminary interview, give them necessary information about the unit but do not overwhelm them with too many details at this time. It is not unusual for relatives and the new resident to be stunned at the sight of so many dementia sufferers under one roof and they are both likely to be upset. A short conversation enables you to sympathise with the new resident and home carer about their feelings of strangeness and apprehension. This also enables you to get to know each other at a closer level. A cup of tea or coffee releases tension.

Take this opportunity to identify any physical or emotional characteristics of the new resident that require special attention and to collect and discuss medication. Encourage questions. The relative, the new resident and staff will all be more comfortable after this sort of introduction to the unit.

### *Unpacking*

The relative will probably appreciate the opportunity to help unpack, put away clothing and belongings, arrange photos and add personal touches.

If a new resident is unaccompanied, do not leave him or her surrounded by luggage, confused, strange and probably frightened, contemplating unfamiliar surroundings alone. Ask them to help you unpack and put away their clothing, and chat while you do so. If staff need to be elsewhere, assign a volunteer for company or take the new arrival with you and come back later.

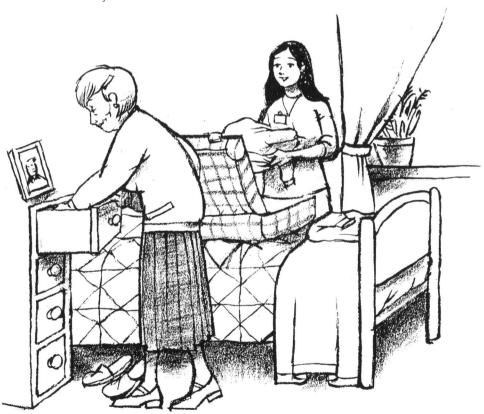

### Introductions

On the first day keep introductions to a minimum.

If the new arrival will be sharing a room, introduce them to room companions, otherwise to one or two residents who live close by or to those with whom they will share a table. The newcomer may already know another resident and you can renew their association. Introduce the relative to another relative.

### Exploring

Invite the relative to stroll around the unit with the newcomer to help them become familiar with the layout. This applies particularly to the relative at this early stage.

The person unaccompanied by a relative or friend may be content to walk around or join in with another resident. It is preferable, however, for a staff member or volunteer to be with a new resident on and off for the first few days to ease confusion and aloneness.

### The end of the first day

Invite the relative to stay for the evening meal and, if possible, wait to settle the new resident into bed for that first night, with the reassurance the relative will return tomorrow. It is better if the relative can stay until the person falls asleep. Where there is no relative or friend a member of staff should stay with the lone resident while he or she drifts off to sleep.

For the first few nights restlessness can be expected, nightmares—often panic—crying out and wandering if the person wakes feeling lost in strange surroundings. Leave a soft light on and make regular checks during the night. Reassure the person who wakens.

The more time the relative or friend can spend with the new resident for the first few days the better will be the adjustment. As the person settles this time can be decreased.

## Adapting to the unit

The new resident will take time to become accustomed to new surroundings and unfamiliar routine.

Some settle more quickly than others but generally it takes from four to six weeks for a person to adapt to life in the unit. The time taken and the manner in which the person adjusts depend on the stage of the illness and the quality of preparation for the move. The newcomer's personality and attitudes of family and staff also affect adjustment.

## Helping to settle

The more personalised attention that can be given, the more quickly the resident will settle. The presence of a relative for as long as possible each day, at meals and bedtime and particularly during difficult periods, reassures the person and facilitates the settling-in process.

Providing short-term accommodation for the spouse who wishes to stay for a few days will help the newcomer adapt more quickly to the unit and ease the separation for both. With communication and understanding this also forms a bond between staff and family.

In most instances it is better for the new resident not to go home, especially overnight, for at least four weeks (unless they have settled earlier). Going back and forth between home and unit shortly after the move may further confuse the person and result in emotional, even violent, outbursts. This impedes the adjustment process for both resident and carer.

## Finding the way around

With repeated 'showing', all but the most severely confused can find their way around in a few days.

Repeatedly help the new resident find their room, pointing out the same markers. Also make them familiar with the layout of the bedroom: clothing drawers, wardrobe, switches, handles and knobs.

You may have to remind new residents to come for meals for the first few days, but if they are able they will soon respond to the cues of kitchen noises or the sound of residents gathering.

## Joining in

It is not a good idea to introduce a newcomer to the group as a whole. To stand him in front of a sea of new faces and announce 'This is a new man, Mr Jones' is likely to embarrass him and make him anxious.

Do not hurry the person to join in the life of the unit. Give newcomers ample time and opportunity to gradually form associations with other residents and find a niche for themselves. Usually the person who is used to a large family or who was an active member of clubs, social and sporting groups joins in quickly. People used to a more solitary life may continue to prefer their own company or a one-to-one relationship.

Where a person enjoys solitary pursuits such as listening to music or watching television, it is better not to deny them lifelong habits by insisting they join group activities. First, however, ascertain that they are not depressed.

## New residents' reactions

Some residents settle in with relative ease, often inventing a reason for being there. Some are even happy in surroundings that are more comfortable than their previous accommodation.

Despair and distress, however, are more usual reactions to moving to a unit and experiencing these feelings is a necessary part of the settling-in process. Even where the transition from home to unit is reasonably smooth, for a time the person will probably be confused and unhappy in the new surroundings.

Invariably, however, the person becomes more confused, memory loss seems worse and the new resident is anxious and fearful. This decreases with time and understanding care.

## Fear of other residents

The newcomer, particularly a woman, is usually afraid of the more assertive or overtly dementing residents and needs constant company and reassurance. Not recognising the characteristics of dementia in themselves, new arrivals may demand, 'What am I doing here with all these mad people?'

Your gentle explanation will usually be accepted: 'No, they aren't mad, they are sick/very confused. And you are not very well.'

## 'I'm in prison'

If someone is not used to a secure environment they often become frustrated, angry or depressed because of the restriction of locked doors and the lack of freedom. The complaint 'I am in prison' or question 'Why are you keeping me in prison?' is not unusual. Respond by saying, 'Yes, it must seem something like a prison to you. But this is a hostel. Look, there's plenty of space for you to walk. Come, I'll walk with you.'

Also do not underestimate the degree of understanding the person may have. A simple explanation such as 'You often get lost in a strange place, and the door being locked keeps you safe' can help.

### *'I'm going home'*

Packing up or otherwise making ready to leave or 'waiting for my daughter—coming to take me home' are common reactions. Diverting the person's attention is probably the best way to deal with this situation. Sometimes just asking the 'going home' person to help replace the clothing in drawers and cupboard is sufficient to divert attention.

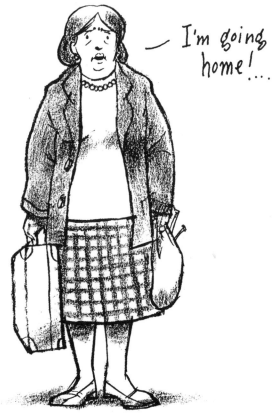

# Blaming relatives

The new resident may vent anger on spouse and family and often refuse to speak to them.

They are accused: 'You put me here so you can take my money' or 'I don't need to be here. I have a very nice home of my own. I can even look after myself'. Nothing will be achieved by explaining that the man refused to eat at home or was lost twice last week. Listen patiently and recognise that the person is telling you that he wants to go home. 'We'll talk about it when your daughter/wife comes' is usually a satisfying answer.

Talk about it with the relative and decide what you are all going to tell the person. For example, everyone will tell him that his wife has hurt her back and can no longer look after him or that he' daughter has moved interstate. Keep as close to the truth as possible because the dementing person, as well as being suspicious, is often shrewd enough to quickly pick up an untruth. Reassuring the person that they are still loved ('You're still our dad') and that someone will visit often is likely to relieve anxiety.

Also do not underestimate the distress that these sorts of accusations have on the family carer: it will help ease the hurt if staff recognise this.

# Extreme emotional reactions

The person may have an excessive emotional reaction a day or two after moving in, when they realise they are not going home. A range of reactions can be expected: determined refusal to eat or cooperate, listlessness, hysteria, aggression, violence, frantic pacing and seeking exits.

Physical and drug restraint are seldom effective, and often increase the intensity of an emotional reaction. Sedation to the extent of continual drowsiness only delays the adjustment process and the person almost always experiences the same reaction when medication is eventually decreased.

Treated with patience and understanding, the newcomer will gradually identify with life in the unit and adjust to the new environment.

*Depression, delusions and hallucinations*

Some new residents suffer deep depression for a time after coming to live in a nursing home or hostel, others develop delusions and hallucinations. These conditions must be properly assessed by a psychiatrist and appropriately treated.

# Relatives' mixed feelings*

The home carer, particularly, will have mixed emotions when the dementing person moves into the residential facility.

Feelings of overwhelming sadness are combined with relief that the burden of caring has been lifted or shared. They worry about the quality of care. Will it be comparable to that at home? Will he or she fret? Will he or she be safe? Will you understand and be considerate of their strange behaviour? The home carer may blame themselves for abandoning the dementing person, even though it is obvious that they can no longer carry on. These feelings are worsened by the dementing person's anger and accusations.

There is a gap in the family carer's life also. They have handed over the carer's role to strangers. The person who has been part of their life for maybe forty years is no longer at home.

The family carer, too, feels abandoned and has great difficulty in adjusting. All family members will have some reaction to residential care and will look to careworkers for understanding.

# Make families welcome

Mutual concerns should be discussed with the family as they arise and the main family member should be taken into staff confidence. Reassure them that they are still needed, that staff can never take their place; that you know a hostel or nursing home can never be quite the same as home but that you will take good care of their relative.

---

*See also section on 'Families' on p. 242.

# THE RESIDENTIAL FACILITY

Aim to create a comfortable homelike environment where the person can be surrounded by personal possessions.

Small, cosy living rooms are preferable. Use screens to divide large rooms.

Avoid the institutional pattern of chairs in rows along walls. Grouped furniture invites social interaction.

Distinctive wall and door colours, cues and markers will help the resident find their way.

Provide opportunities to keep in touch with the real world:

—verandahs overlooking houses, streets and parks

—open windows to let in the outside sounds and smells

—a public telephone to maintain a link with home and family

The aim is to create an environment where the person lives in a comfortable homelike atmosphere surrounded by personal belongings.

Units vary from small, specially built cottages to cavernous institutions. With imaginative renovation, however, even a large institution can become a comfortable and more personal place to live.

Mobile residents should preferably be accommodated apart from those who are frail or chairbound. This allows for a lifestyle that is more suited to them. It also protects those who cannot defend themselves from the irritation of people wandering into their rooms, pilfering belongings or on occasions attacking them.

## Personal furniture and possessions

Encourage the person to bring as much personal furniture as space and management will allow to enhance the impression of home. If it is not possible to bring the person's bed, a chair, bedcover or cushion is comforting. Familiar curtains at the window can give much satisfaction. For a few, a personal radio and television set provide choice of entertainment and a means of sharing with friends in their own rooms.

Photographs, ornaments, a favourite handbag or much loved coat or apron are familiar and comforting and add to a homelike atmosphere. A scrapbook with personal mementoes, such as theatre programs, tickets and newspaper clippings, also provides memory cues for some people.

# Bedrooms

Everybody needs a space to call one's own, preferably a single room with a door. Locks are not a good idea, as more often than not keys are lost and staff are faced with picking locks or climbing through windows.

Shared rooms should be divided into equal spaces (curtains screening only the bed space are not enough) and institutional wards should be partitioned into single rooms of adequate size.

### *Furniture and possessions*

Each room or space should contain a wardrobe, dressing table or chest of drawers, and shelves for ornaments. Ample wall-space will accommodate pictures and photographs. Where the person is likely to destroy or does not have personal belongings, a bright poster on the wall supplies colour and interest. Brown paper bags for rubbish are better than open bins or wastepaper baskets, which can be removed to personal rooms or mistaken for toilet bowls.

If the resident is chairbound, it defeats the purpose to place photographs and personal possessions on the wall behind the bed. Turn the bed and chair around so that they can see them.

### *Flooring and curtains*

Where incontinence is a problem, a washable floor covering is essential and sill-length curtains are less likely to be soiled than those reaching to the floor. Floor mats and rugs should not be used as residents may trip on them and fall.

# Bathrooms

Individual bathrooms can be colourful and furnished as tastefully as those in a private home. Because most individual shower rooms allow for wheelchair access they tend to be unattractive and impersonal. One dementia unit decorated ensuites with a wallpaper border around the wall below the ceiling.

Where facilities are shared, most people prefer to have separate bathrooms and toilets for men and women.

# Living rooms

Living rooms should be comfortable and homely. Small, cosy rooms are preferable to large ones. The person who is watching television resents sharing the room with a bingo game. The chatty craft group does not want to be deafened by community singing. Having a piano and two television sets in one room is not a good idea.

Relatives and friends will appreciate a private space for a visit with the resident. If you have only one small living room, are there waste spaces at the end of corridors or tucked-away nooks? Even small spaces can be furnished attractively and used for a variety of purposes: visiting, reading, sharing a meal or afternoon tea with a friend.

Divide large living rooms with screens. In dining rooms, stack chairs and tables and use the area for activities between meals. Maybe the dining room can double as a television room?

## *Chairs*

Comfort and ease of rising is paramount in the design of all chairs. The design should incorporate two solid arms, a seat of a comfortable height and floor space underneath the seat. Where cane or wicker chairs are used, use padded arm cushions to protect frail skin from injury. Vinyl upholstery is preferable to cloth as it is easily cleaned. If laundry facilities can cope, bright loose covers and washable cushions are attractive and cosy.

## *Wall units*

Wall units and sideboards are preferable to enclosed wall cupboards. One hostel displays residents' treasures on the top shelves of a wall unit in a much used small sitting room. There residents can see their more valuable vases and ornaments brought from home. Even a silver tea service and a large crystal vase.

In this same hostel, pot plants grow happily near windows or glass doors and provide interest and activity for the gardener. However, where pot plants and flower containers are included in the living room decor, place them out of reach of the person who likes to pick and weed or examine roots to check their growth.

### Furniture arrangement

Furniture arranged in small groups invites social interaction. Plenty of space between groupings allows some privacy and decreases bruising and falls as residents try to weave their way through tables and chairs. Occasional tables with magazines and one or two easy chairs placed around the unit provide a quiet place to sit, and act as a distraction from walking.

Tables should be round as sharp corners often cause injury. They should seat four for dining and two or more tables can be pulled together for craft and other activities.

Avoid the institutional pattern of chairs in rows along walls.

## Mirrors

Full-length, impact-resistant mirrors assist grooming and appearance, and the person's image reinforces a sense of identity. Mirrors on exit doors reduce attempts to go through them.

Very occasionally there will be a resident who objects to 'the person in the mirror' and becomes frightened or wants to attack. This person could be accommodated as far away as possible from the mirror. Or if each room is fitted with a mirror, cover it or obscure it with furniture or a soluble paint such as the white spray that is used for Christmas decoration. Check to see that the paint is not toxic.

## Cues to location

Cues or markers will help the person find his or her way around. Some suggestions are:

- distinctive wall and door colours;
- pictures and photographs placed at strategic points along the route;
- nameplates and illustrations, for example on toilet and in bathroom, television room and dining room (avoid commercial symbols as they are are sometimes confusing);
- bedroom doors each of a different colour;
- a name plate, small picture or photograph of the person's spouse or family on the bedroom door;
- even a number on the bedroom door, where there are several doors opening off a corridor.

Certain signs such as 'Exit' are a regulatory safety requirement in some states. However, arrows and signs such as 'Exit', 'Out', 'Up to kiosk', 'Down to car park' and 'Stairs' also act as cues for wanderers and, where they cannot be avoided, extra care needs to be exercised with determined 'escapologists'.

## Links with the outside world

The design of any residential facility should provide opportunities for the resident to maintain contact with the world outside. High windows and solid walls emphasise the feeling of imprisonment that is strong in some residents.

### *Looking out*

Residents like to see the outside world. Windows and shatterproof glass doors should allow views of nearby houses, roads, traffic and footpaths where people come and go.

> Picture a comfortable unit with windows and doors looking over walled gardens, a comfortable recreation room and television tuned to the morning program. Breakfast is about to be served. Yet waiting residents cluster around the foyer or walk in the garden near the front gate, now and again peering over the fence.

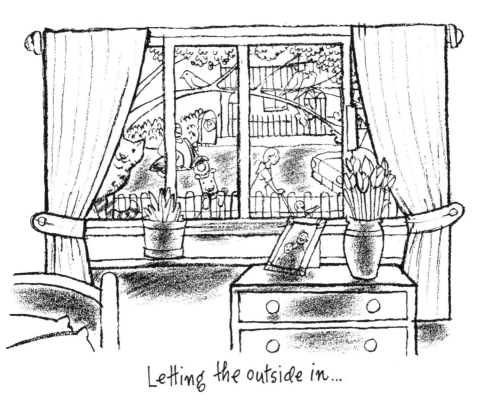

Letting the outside in...

An equally comfortable and stimulating dementia ward in a psychiatric hospital has a large wire front gate. Patients gather around it at every opportunity.

———

Residents spend happy times on the verandah and in the sunroom of a hostel designed to overlook the local school yard next door. Their enjoyment at watching is unmistakable as they chatter amongst themselves about the activities of the children below.

In each of these scenarios, the residents choose to be in the place where they can watch the world go by.

## *Sounds and smells*

Sounds and smells are an important part of our normal environment. It may not be possible to reproduce the sounds of the harbour or the smells of the farm or city but we need not restrict the person to the noise of trolleys, rattling china and the smell of disinfectant.

Flowers bring fragrance to the unit. The smells of cooking seeping through the open kitchen door, coffee brewing, rain on hot earth, cosmetics or even furniture polish are all familiar aromas.

Open the windows. Let the sounds of the world in. The distant singer, the dog barking, bird songs in the evening, the calls of children and the occasional screech of brakes will make the unit seem more like home.

## *Telephones*

The ability to use a telephone is retained for a long time and represents a valuable link to family and friends. A coin-operated phone can be installed to be used as the person wishes. On occasions staff may have to help with finding numbers or dialling. The phone can also be programmed to receive incoming calls so relatives can ring in on the public phone, thus easing the traffic on unit phones.

Check with relatives about the resident's use of the phone. Some, particularly those who are anxious or who have no immediate memory, may ring out repeatedly to the same number with the same message. As a last resort, excessive phoning can be controlled by limiting the daily number of coins.

# LIFE IN THE RESIDENTIAL FACILITY

The foremost consideration must be the person's need and right to be treated with dignity.

The foundation of a satisfactory lifestyle is good physical care, trained staff working as a team and a flexible routine.

When you are planning, take into account the person's previous lifestyle.

Involve families as part of the working team.

**Make life enjoyable. Encourage fun and laughter and wherever possible adultness and individuality.**

**Aim to retain the person's level of functioning, independence and self-identity for as long as possible.**

**Try not to over-protect the person.**

# The resident's daily life

Good physical care, a flexible routine and staff working as a team are the foundation on which to build a satisfactory daily life for the resident.

Attitudes that encourage adultness and individuality, socialising and keeping in touch with the real world improve the quality of the person's lifestyle.

On the other hand, it is difficult if not impossible to create an enjoyable life for the person who is over-sedated, overwhelmed by too much stimulation or in a situation where management procedures take precedence over people needs.

## *Routine*

Routine is the regular arrangement of unit procedure, a timetable that operates twenty-four hours a day, seven days a week: meals, bathing, activities, rest at the same time each day, regular outings and entertainment.

A routine structures the day, helps to balance the person's confusion and indecision and stimulates anticipation of enjoyable events. The routine must be flexible enough to allow for personal choices if you are to encourage people with dementia to maintain as much control over their lives as they are capable of.

In some nursing homes and hostels, late breakfasts are available when residents choose to sleep in, and a cup of tea and a chat when they are sleepless. A choice of activity is allowed: to sit in the garden rather than to play bingo; to watch television rather than to do craft; to stay home from an excursion to rest or walk at will.

Above all, flexibility allows the person to retain individuality.

## *Avoid regimentation*

In a regimented unit, residents do everything together as a group. Lives are organised from getting-up to bedtime. Residents have to bath, eat, sleep, come in and go out to suit shift changes or other institutional rules and requirements. Their own wishes are seldom taken into consideration. Emphasis is on what 'they' have forgotten rather than what the individual person is still able to do. There is little or no choice. Regimentation is preferred in some units because it is considered to be quicker and more efficient to 'do for' the resident rather than encourage independence.

Regimentation stereotypes residents and the conformity expected is very often at the level of the lowest functioning resident, causing frustration to those who are able to operate at a higher level. A few residents adapt quickly to the demands of the regimented unit but many vigorously resist attempts to make them conform and they struggle for their independence. They may have catastrophic reactions. To avoid stress, however, a person will eventually behave in the way that is expected of them. The consequence of this is the loss of the little control that they have over their life. Skills are prematurely forgotten and the person becomes submissive and apathetic. This is often called 'institutional behaviour'* and is not associated with the person's dementia.

Institutional behaviour can be modified and sometimes reversed. Provide stimulating surroundings and activities and encourage the person to be appropriately independent.

> The occupational therapist arranges a tea-party for ten women in the dementia unit. Apart from reaching for a cake and examining the empty cups, they ignore the prettily set table. Accustomed to tea served ready to drink, they have forgotten about teapots, sugar basins and milk jugs, even to the point where they do not know that spoons are for stirring.
>
> Regular tea-parties and eventually a change in procedure to allow more independence restores these and other unused skills.

---

*Also called institutionalisation.

# Staff

Dementing people need to see familiar faces; staff changes can be unsettling. In units where the working atmosphere is pleasant and staff are recognised as valued members of the organisation, staff turnover is low. However, because of the stress on staff of interacting with dementia for long periods, staff will need a change of employment from time to time.

When the staff member's move from the unit is imminent, it should be discussed with the residents some time beforehand. This allows the residents to become used to the idea and work through their separation anxieties. A special farewell party, such as a special afternoon tea or a cake at lunchtime, is a good idea to finalise the worker's relationship with the residents.

## *Training*

All workers who are employed to care for people with dementia require some training in caring for dementia residents, especially in communication and relationship skills. The knowledge gained gives a competence in difficult work and adds to staff members' feelings of self-esteem.

## *The team*

A team consists of everyone who works in the dementia unit. Relatives are an important part of the team. A team will only work well or even work at all if there is continuing and open communication amongst its members. There are a number of ways this can be facilitated.

---

**Working together as a team promotes harmony and satisfaction for staff and a contented unit overall.**

---

## *Sharing information*

Sharing information allows the team to work out solutions to problems and plan a consistent approach to residents. The likelihood of duplication and confusion is reduced: Mrs Joyner is not taken on the bus trip when she has an appointment with the dentist.

Practical information, such as appointments, family visits and change of medication, can be shared by communication books or boards. Short weekly or fortnightly meetings are also a means of sharing information and discussing plans and problems and they can save hours otherwise spent in sorting out tangles.

### Sharing tasks

While each discipline in the team has its own expertise, many tasks, such as feeding, walking, chatting and activities can be shared. It is just as effective for the domestic worker to reminisce with the resident while cleaning the room as it is for the diversional therapist to conduct a structured reminiscence group.

# Involving relatives

A satisfactory relationship between families and staff promotes understanding, reduces conflict and benefits everyone concerned.

### Seek advice from relatives

Relatives, particularly the home carer, are the single most important resource for staff caring for the dementing person. They have an intimate knowledge of the resident, having cared for them during the long progression of the illness. They can provide valuable guidelines for management of physical caring, response to emotional behaviour and provide solutions to problems you might encounter. Seek their advice.

> Mrs Aston disrupts the life of the unit, calling out, throwing magazines and attacking staff. After her husband is consulted she is again placed on the routine that had been worked out over some time at home between her husband and her doctor.
>
> She is woken at five o'clock, showered and then allowed to drift off to sleep to the sounds of her favourite classical music. After breakfast in bed at ten, Mrs Aston is ready to start the day. At the first sign of disruptive behaviour, she is taken to her room to listen to her cassette player.

## Relatives can help with caring

Many residential facilities are understaffed and relatives can provide invaluable assistance as volunteers. In one unit, part of the caring is carried out by relatives who are welcomed as members of the team. At ten o'clock a few husbands and wives arrive by bus. Until three o'clock they walk, talk, change and feed their 'own' resident. Acting as volunteers they help staff by including other residents in walks or discussions, sorting clothes and supervising activities.

This assistance is invaluable to residential facilities, many of which are understaffed and where a proportion of residents have no relatives or friends to visit.

## Keeping families informed

Too often when the resident moves to a nursing home or hostel, families feel they have given up all rights to their relative. Many of those who visit infrequently do so because they do not feel welcome. One way of overcoming this feeling is to keep them informed of the resident's doings during a friendly chat about how the resident, say, enjoyed the outing or community singing; how they remembered words of songs, achieved part of a task or was involved in a funny incident.

## Family groups

A family group is a valuable part of the life of the unit. It helps relatives feel as though they have a place and gives them status. The support that members gain from each other not only eases their anxiety but relieves pressure on staff.

Families also feel more confident and safe when a request for information or a complaint comes from the group as a whole. Individually, they may be reluctant to complain in case they are thought to be a nuisance or their relative is disadvantaged in some way. Not wanting to appear ignorant or stupid, they may hesitate to seek much needed information.

## Relatives can suggest improvements

Some nursing homes and dementia units encourage family groups to make suggestions about the services offered. By having regular meetings in the unit, and sometimes with a member of staff included, relatives also develop an appreciation of the work of staff and the difficulties that are experienced from day to day. Mutual trust and a happier unit is the result.

# A normal style of life

For the daily life of residents to be satisfactory and enjoyable it must have meaning to them as individuals and resemble as far as possible the lives elderly people live in their own homes.

In order to pursue a normal style of life, the person needs opportunities to do familiar things, play out life-roles and engage in retained interests. The personal profile and functional assessment, personal possessions and discussions with relatives provide information as to how you can achieve this.

---

**To help promote a satisfactory lifestyle you will need to know:**

◆ **the person's interests:**

 —gardening, farming, woodwork, sewing

 —golf, cricket, football

 —crosswords, quizzes

 —singing, music, television, radio;

◆ **what the person is able to do and what they *like* to do;**

◆ **what they like to talk about;**

◆ **the person's beliefs and values;**

◆ **what they enjoy and what irritates them.**

When you obtain this sort of information you will begin to see the resident, not as just another person with dementia you have the responsibility of caring for but as the person they were before they were affected by dementia. Remember Louise, the lobbyist, in Chapter 5?

---

### Feeling at home

With your help, the resident gradually becomes involved in the life of the unit and develops a feeling of 'belonging'. They relate more and more to other residents and begin to trust staff. Some develop a strong sense of ownership for their rooms or personal spaces. In the sitting room time may be spent in a preferred place or the resident may claim a special chair as they did at home.

## Friendships

A resident may make a close friend. Most friendships are formed between people who are functioning at the same level or whose behaviour has the same characteristics. Those who retain a social veneer tend to form groups or one-to-one friendships. They sit together, enjoy frequent 'chats' and join the same activities. Walkers seek each other's company. Observe them hand in hand, strolling around the unit.

Similar interests or background do not seem to influence greatly the forming of friendships. In fact, a person may be irritated by someone who has the same interests but who functions at a lower level. Sometimes close friendships are based on mistaken identity or someone who looks like a friend or a loved one from the past.

Friendships suffer stresses and strains. Petty jealousies and disagreements usually resolve themselves but at times staff may have to intervene.

### Relatives may not approve

Occasionally relatives may query the wisdom of a close friendship, especially if a member of the opposite sex is involved.

> Kathleen 'adopts' Roger and refers to him as 'my husband' or sometimes as 'my friend'. She fusses over him and feeds him when he can no longer handle a spoon or fork.
>
> Her family objects to the friendship when the two are found lying together on his bed. When they are parted, they fret. The friendship happily continues after a round table discussion with both families.

### Identifying with a friend

It is not unusual for the person with dementia to be sensitive to the feelings of a friend and on occasions to feel it necessary to interpret these to staff. The friend may even be aggressively defended if the person perceives them to be unfairly treated or in danger.

### Providing company

The person with dementia appears to enjoy company more than any other pastime.

> In a large institution several people with dementia were asked: 'Who helps you the most?' The answer: '...because he has time to listen.'
>
> Sit and walk with the resident; listen and talk to them. Look at magazines together or join with them in some activity.

A voluntary companion is a valuable resource for one-to-one interaction with a person who enjoys the company of another.

## Fun and laughter

Inject liveliness into the daily life of the unit by providing moments of fun and laughter. The person with dementia invariably retains a characteristic sense of humour. Exploit this.

Laugh with the residents. The person is often aware that what he or she says or does is silly or irrational and will see the funny side.

Always take care to laugh with the person, not at them.

## Toilet articles and clothing

Each person should have his or her own toilet articles and cosmetics. If electric razors or other toilet articles are likely to be misused, keep them in the locked part of the wardrobe or in a locked drawer.

A person should always wear their own clothes. Drip-dry and unshrinkable garments are preferable where incontinence is a problem. Tracksuits are better than trousers which require dry cleaning. Some facilities prefer dresses and slips that can be arranged to either side when sitting to cut down on the number of changes. Keep a set of going-out clothes for special occasions. Clothing provided by the unit should be used only in emergencies, and then only briefly.

Make sure everyone is adequately clothed for prevailing weather conditions. Some may not be sensitive to heat and cold, or if they are, the brain may not say 'Put on your jumper' or 'Throw off the blanket'. Outside in the warmer months, sun hats and sunscreen cream are a necessity. Take special care to protect those who are taking chlorpromazine (Largactil).

# Appearance

A neat appearance and good grooming enhance the person's self-image and self-esteem. Help the person to select clothes for the day if necessary. Encourage women to use make-up if it has been their habit and men to shave daily. Regular visits to the hairdresser and an occasional manicure will add to the self-image. Use mirrors to confirm appearance and offer praise for 'looking nice'.

# Visitors

Encourage family and friends to visit as often as they can comfortably manage.

Visits from children are a welcome diversion and usually create great excitement amongst residents. Children's visits are better limited to short periods, ending before they become tired, bored, exuberant and noisy. And not too many children at once.

### No visitors?

If the resident has no visitors, try to find a companion or regular visitor by contacting the local church, ethnic group or Returned Servicemen's League, whichever is applicable. Some community aid groups have a list of visitors trained to relate to people with dementia.

# Pets

Someone who is withdrawn or has difficulty in relating to staff and other residents may benefit from the companionship of a pet animal.

If the pet is to be a dog, make sure that it is old enough and wise enough to avoid the foot of an unfriendly resident. The group Pets as Therapy will visit with a suitable dog and Guide Dogs for the Blind or animal shelters such as the RSPCA often have dogs that are suitable as permanent pets.

# Taking risks

The need to protect residents from harm and allow them to take some risks is sometimes a fine balance. Apart from having a duty of care, staff are understandably reluctant to expose residents to situations where there is a risk of harm, in case of accusations of negligence. On the other hand over-protection deprives the resident of many pleasurable experiences.

## *Over-protection*

❝ The nursing unit manager makes new rules for Ward X, the dementia ward. Patients are strictly supervised at all times, activity and leisure materials are locked away except during organised sessions. Brooms, knitting, craft material, movable articles and some personal possessions are confiscated in case they are used harmfully. Walking areas are restricted to a small section, only to be used at set times.

Before shift changes, patients are contained in one room where they can be watched while paperwork is brought up to date.

The level of anxiety in the ward rises and some residents react with agitation and aggression. With others, apathy increases. ❞

## *Discuss risk taking with relatives*

Where there is an element of risk, discuss the circumstances with the relative and ask for written consent for the resident to participate.

Sometimes a relative will insist that the resident be physically or chemically restrained for reasons of safety, even though you may explain that this is not a desirable practice. In cases such as this, it is advisable to obtain written authority from the relative even before you seek advice as to the best course of action.

# KEEPING OCCUPIED

The person with dementia needs opportunities to engage in activities they enjoy.

Allow opportunities for the resident to pursue a chosen pastime. Activity does not have to be limited to structured sessions.

Avoid overstimulating the person with too much activity. The resident needs time out occasionally to sit and contemplate or just to sit.

Structured activities should cater for adult interests and be within the person's capabilities.

Allow for short concentration span and impaired eyesight and hearing.

Design a balanced program—a mix of physical and intellectual activity, craft, entertainment and excursions.

Be prepared to abandon or modify your activity program if residents are reluctant to participate or if they tire. If the person refuses to participate, coax, do not force.

Occasional noisy activities are fun. Continuous din is annoying.

## Occupying the resident

Keeping residents occupied is important in order to enhance the quality of their lives and to retain their interest and skills while ever it is possible.

Some residents are able to occupy themselves reasonably well—women in particular. Some will successfully fill their days, often sitting and 'chatting' to staff or other residents or enjoying visits with relatives or someone else's visitors. They will sort and fold and 'tidy' drawers and dust and polish and put away. In between, they may stroll around with a friend; they may choose to join excursions or attend a concert or participate in bingo or singing. In fact, given the opportunity, some women seem to live a full and active life for quite a long time.

Male residents seem less likely to occupy themselves except for occasional short periods. This is probably due to the fact that many traditional men's skills cannot be used in a residential facility. In addition, many men seem to be in a more progressed stage of the disease when they move to a hostel or nursing home and have lost their ability to carry out an activity independently.

If the person with dementia does not have enough occupation they will appear to deteriorate rapidly, becoming listless and apathetic, sitting or wandering aimlessly, often into other people's rooms to rummage and pilfer. You should provide plenty of opportunities for residents to engage in a range of activities, and participate and supervise when necessary.

# Get the most from each day

'The aim is to try to get the most enjoyment out of each day. It is important to take [one] day at a time, do [one] activity at a time, and to stimulate the person without overwhelming him or her. For some, [ten] minutes may be sufficient for an activity, for others, an hour or [two] is appreciated. The aim of the activity is to try and stimulate parts of the brain not affected by the illness and derive enjoyment from the activity.'*

# Free choice of activity

Keeping the person occupied should not be limited to structured activity sessions.

Do not lock away all activity material overnight or from Friday afternoon until Monday morning. Do provide an assortment of activity material for residents to fill in moments during the day.

You may need to help with the activity of the person's choice.

---

* Professor Henry Brodaty, Academic Department of Psychogeriatrics, University of New South Wales/Prince Henry Hospital, Sydney.

## Magazines

Scatter magazines and newspapers in living areas. Men enjoy 'reading' trade, technical and sports magazines and business reports.

Magazines have the tendency to disappear rather quickly, so you will need a source of supply. Relatives, friends and local service clubs can usually provide a range of reading material.

## Books

If the person has some comprehension and likes to read, make arrangements with the mobile lending library to call weekly. Large-print books are available from most libraries. Organisations such as the Royal Blind Society lend talking books for the person who has impaired eyesight.

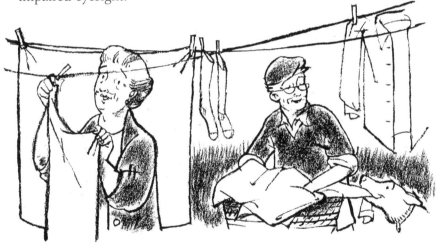

## Domestic chores

Not every resident is interested in domestic chores. Others happily dust, polish and sweep on and off all day. Some like to help with the washing-up, gardening or repairs. Others accompany staff and assist with bed making, tidying, emptying rubbish, arranging flowers, watering pot plants and folding laundry. Helping staff with tasks around the unit gives people a sense of belonging and puts a purpose into their day.

Leave brooms, dustpans and brushes, and dusters where they are visible and accessible and encourage the gardener to weed or dig. If landscaped plants are at risk of destruction, provide a special place for the gardener to work.

## Television and radio

In their own homes many residents watch favourite television programs. Morning variety and midday serials are popular as well as many evening shows such as quizzes and serials. Foreign-language and travel programs are interesting to residents from other countries and those who have toured overseas.

The resident may prefer to watch television with friends in the privacy of their room or to watch on the unit television switched to favoured programs. Make sure the chairbound person is not left in front of the television set for long periods.

Personal radios and cassette players allow the person who is interested in music, opera or other familiar programs to indulge those interests.

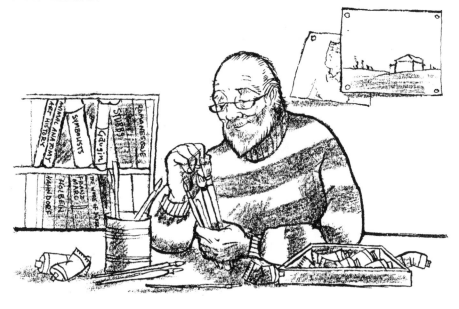

## *Other individual interests*

Many residents have personal interests.

> Each day the artist who can no longer paint sorts through his brushes, caressing each one; then he carefully packs them away until next time.
>
> ———
>
> One man regularly scans his photograph album, while another conscientiously writes down columns of numbers as the volunteer calls them.
>
> ———
>
> Each time the two women sit, they extract their knitting from carry-bags; knit and chat.
>
> ———
>
> Another resident 'plays' with the pack of cards he carries in his pocket. Sometimes he joins with three others to 'play' bridge or poker. It does not matter that there is no sense to the game. They enjoy it.

## *Reminiscing*

We all like to remember pleasant experiences and relationships. None more so than the person with dementia. Nostalgia or recalling past experiences and relationships is often spontaneous. Two or more residents will chat together about past events, each recalling their own memories.

Remembering events of long ago or discussing a recent pleasant experience need not be limited to structured group discussions. Staff can sit with the person and look at photographs together, ask how he met his wife, their wedding and their family. Do not persist if the person is reluctant to discuss their life, or is distressed by an unpleasant memory.

Some people prefer to recall more recent events. They may remember the family visiting yesterday, the picnic in the park last week or how much they enjoyed the community singing. Being able to talk about the present is often more enjoyable than talking about the past.

### Just sitting

Like everyone else, people with dementia need to have time to themselves. Some spend time just sitting or enjoying a rest on the bed for an hour or two.

# Structured activity

Activities should:

◆ cater for adult interests. Many feel patronised if they are asked to participate in what they perceive as childish activity. They may refuse or leave after a minute or two. At best they will tolerate being included.
◆ have broad aims such as enjoyment, enhancing feelings of importance, socialising and keeping fit. The activity is a means of achieving the aim.
◆ be within the person's abilities. Success is more likely when one part of an activity is attempted rather than the whole. Keep the risk of failure to a minimum.

### Designing the program

The design of the activity program should allow for a mix of craft, physical and intellectual activity, outings and entertainment interspersed with quiet or free-choice times. In some facilities the stated aim of an activities program is to keep the residents occupied and out of their rooms during the day. This means that residents, to meet the requirements of administration, are often forced into taking part in activities that do not interest them or that they dislike.

*Activity programs must fit the needs of the residents.* Where a facility's administration designs an activities program purely to keep residents occupied and out of their rooms, the program will not be effective.

### *Flexibility*

Activity programs need to be flexible. Be prepared to modify or abandon an activity that residents try to escape from. Residents often do not want to participate in a particular activity or at the scheduled time. They may have no interest in a particular activity. They may tire easily. On bad days in the unit, residents are often reluctant to be involved in any activity. They should not be forced if they refuse after encouragement and coaxing.

Display the timetable where it can be seen by residents, families and staff. Some residents are interested to check on a favourite activity and will pass the information on to others.

## Aim to maintain skills and interests

Design activities so that they help to maintain the person's skills for as long as possible. Find out what his or her interests were at home and cater for these as well as current interests. Remember to encourage the use of the person's retained abilities.

Make allowances for memory loss and confusion, poor judgment and difficulties in recognising objects and knowing their use. Also make allowances for the following.

### *Sight and hearing*

Many people have impaired vision. Some have no peripheral vision (tunnel vision), which means they see only directly to the front. Others can see but cannot interpret what they see.

Make sure the person hears and understands what you are saying.

### *Concentration*

The ability to concentrate differs from person to person: some are capable of paying attention for an hour or more; others not at all. The more meaningful and appropriate the activity is for the person, the longer their interest will be maintained.

 Mr Errol quickly lost interest in all the activities in the unit, unable to concentrate for more than a few minutes. One day the diversional therapist brought in bundles of small branches and string for use in a creative craft activity. Mr Errol took a great interest in weaving shapes from this material and could be found on most days creating mobiles and 'sculptures' from the material. His aimless wandering ceased and he would concentrate on his activity for hours.

Concentration may fluctuate and this will contribute to inconsistent performance. Someone may be able to do an activity one day but not the next, depending on their concentration at that particular time. Do not persist with the activity. It is better to let the person rest or encourage them to go for a stroll.

### One activity can be performed

Despite confusion and memory loss, someone may still be able to perform one or two activities or tasks quite independently.

Prudence has little understanding of what goes on around her. Left alone she just sits. Yet for two hours each day, she uses an electric machine and sews straight seams.

### Part of an activity can be performed

A complete task or activity may be beyond the capability of a person, but some part of it may be manageable.

With supervision several people can set a table: one is responsible for placing peppers and salts, one for setting knives, another for spoons, and so on. In a cookery group, one person peels bananas, while another hulls the strawberries. Mr Lawson whips the cream (watch that he does not eat it by the handful!), Mr Han sprinkles the icing sugar and Mrs Pringle enjoys setting out the pretty china bowls.

# Physical activities

Physical activities are fun. They also help the person to retain an awareness of where the body parts are and to exploit the sense of rhythm.

## *Exercise*

Exercise is essential for health and helps to promote sleep. Most residents will join in morning and evening strolls outside the unit, morning exercise groups and soft ball throwing. Those who walk for many hours each day will have sufficient exercise.

Some units have regular weekly visits to the local pool for those residents who like to swim.

## *Dancing*

The dementing person usually retains a keen sense of rhythm. Most will enjoy dancing, doing the conga or simply swaying to music.

# Intellectual activities

Often the person who is confused and has little memory will enjoy and is successful in activities that require mental skills. Blackboard games, word-building and matching countries and towns, recognition of pictures are entered into with animation and crossword puzzles are attempted with enthusiasm.

### *Link discussion with activity*

Do you find discussion groups hard to get started and to keep going? Try weaving the discussion around an activity. You will need to take an active role by encouraging each person to take part in the discussion. Even the person with little speech can enjoy the interaction.

On a bus trip there are many sights, sounds and smells that trigger memories; a house, a fence or a tree or flower may remind someone of their own home and garden, and they can be encouraged to talk about it. Invariably others will want to tell about their houses and gardens, sometimes vying to outdo each other with their stories.

 Every time the bus passes a garden with a camellia bush, Miss P. tells the story of her 'beautiful pink camellia tree', which she says is in her front garden. She tells how she has to go out each morning and rake the flowers from under the tree. Other residents respond and sympathise with her for 'all that hard work you have to do every day'.

Food preparation and cooking are activities that seem to arouse interest and stimulate reminiscences of both men and women. Preparation of other meals at other times are remembered, for example mother cooking—even the particular way she beat the eggs and sugar, or chilled the pastry. Favourite recipes may be recalled and family anecdotes recounted. Once the discussion is moving along, it is possible for it to become spontaneous, and at times to awaken many and varied memories.

### Craft and homemaking

Participants in craft work can see and handle the results of their efforts.

Suitable craft and homemaking activities are numerous and most can be broken down into simple steps. In one unit cushion making is a source of occupation and enjoyment. Both men and women participate by cutting, stitching and stuffing. Cushions quickly disappear into private rooms and onto beds.

### Entertainment

Show films and videos occasionally. Films should have movement rather than dialogue and the content should be colourful, familiar or attractive to the residents. Musicals, ballet, variety concerts and military tattoos are all popular.

You might find interest waning if the film is too long. Consider showing half, or less. View the film with the residents. Films often awaken memories and stimulate discussion.

### Music

The person's appreciation of music and sense of rhythm usually survive longer than intellectual functions.

A CD or cassette player is a necessity in every unit. Play music that is familiar to residents; some will like musical comedy and jazz but pop music from the seventies on is seldom tolerated. The classical music lover will enjoy videos of symphony concerts and opera.

Music if playing continuously can become irritating, people often becoming agitated. A resident may try to turn it off, often damaging the player in the process.

### Group singing

Most residents will enjoy singing, while others tap or nod or sway in recognition of a familiar tune. Tunes and lyrics preferred by this generation are usually those associated with the person's younger days, particularly those from World War II and after.

A selection of suitable tapes and CDs is available. Try those featuring Vera Lynn, Bing Crosby, Glen Miller, Perry Como, Gracie Fields, Paul Robeson, the Andrews Sisters, Mitch Miller and his band. Many of these tunes will also be familiar to people of European non-English-speaking backgrounds and they will often sing along using the words of their native language. Songs such as 'Daisy, Daisy' and 'It's a long way to Tipperary' and other folk songs of that era are still enjoyed by some, even though they belong to a generation that has all but died out and are often unfamiliar to people of non-English-speaking cultures.

### Concerts

Do you have a local ballet school or children's choir willing to perform occasionally for residents?

Musical societies and church choirs will sometimes come to the unit and there are groups that receive government funding to provide entertainment for nursing homes and hostels. You might find a volunteer who will come regularly to play an instrument or bring records for a musical hour.

# Noise

Noisy, lively activities in small doses are fun, but a high level of continuous noise exasperates both staff and residents. Loud and continuous music is as undesirable as no music. Combined with alarms, the babble of voices, metallic bangings from the kitchen and the hum of cleaners and polishers, it will distress everybody.

Restrict noisy activities to rooms that can be closed off. Play music only when residents will enjoy it. Conduct craft and quiet groups away from distractions. Provide quiet places where the residents can get away from noise.

Change the routine so that noisy activities take place at different times of the day: for example, do not vacuum at breakfast-time. Arrange for residents to be in the garden or walking outside the unit when the noise level is high.

# Excursions

Going out adds variety to the residents' lives and keeps them in touch with the outside world. Keep daily excursions short and simple: a weekly bus trip, morning tea in the park or a picnic. Staff also benefit from a change of scenery.

Do not change the venue every outing. Residents tend to prefer and look forward to visiting familiar places and recognise landmarks joyfully.

## Holidays

Holidays have been arranged with various degrees of success for groups of residents from a few nursing homes and hostels. Selection of appropriate residents to take part needs great care, excluding anyone who is unable to tolerate change or feels unsafe outside the confines of the residential facility. These people are unlikely to benefit from the holiday, often having catastrophic reactions to strange surroundings. However, staff have reported that most residents thoroughly enjoy themselves, while the staff often come back in varying stages of exhaustion!

## Going to church

If the resident was accustomed to going to church, synagogue or mosque and still can, make arrangements for attendance at religious services. If the family is unable to accompany the resident, a member of the congregation may agree to pick them up and return them to the unit.

## *Family outings*

Encourage family outings.

However, large or prolonged family gatherings or outings, such as attending public concerts or the ballet, are not always a good idea. It is preferable for the resident to stay a short time, otherwise she or he may become overtired, overstimulated and confused. Anxiety or fear may precipitate a catastrophic reaction.

Sometimes an overnight stay at home is possible. However, when it fails families often feel they are to blame. They will battle through a turbulent night rather than return the person to the unit. Prepare them for possible failure, emphasising that it is better to bring the resident back.

On return to the unit, the resident may be disturbed, sometimes having a catastrophic reaction.

> From the beginning, Mr Kent visited his wife each day and would pick her up on Friday night to stay at home till Sunday evening. When she arrived back at the unit there would always be a catastrophic reaction and it took a day or two for staff to settle her down. The family shared their concern with the staff about Mrs Kent's behaviour at home and the effect it was having on their father. Mr Kent insisted that he wanted her with him as much as possible.
>
> One day he took his wife to the shopping mall. She became violent, throwing articles from the open shelves and screaming at the sales people.
>
> Following a plan made with staff, Mrs Kent was not taken out for six weeks and she returned to her normal quiet self. After that Mr Kent would take her out occasionally for a few hours and after a time he gradually extended her visits to a night at home. There were no more outbursts.

## *Reluctance to go out*

Occasionally a resident develops a fear of leaving the security of the unit. You may be able to persuade them to do so and the outing will be enjoyed. On the other hand, someone may comply, but once outside panic.

Do not insist. Recognise that the resident feels safe in the unit. Next time they may go without protest.

If the fear persists you may be able to help the person overcome it by gradually getting them used to leaving the unit. Over a period of days (it may take a week or two) increase the distance the person goes from the unit in gradual steps by taking them:

1   just outside
2   for a walk in the garden or the street
3   to sit in the car or bus
4   for a short drive
5   for a whole outing

Should the person resist any one step, do not proceed. Next day or after a few days start again from the first step until they willingly participate in each step. The fear will eventually be overcome.

# FAMILIES

**Every member of the family is affected by dementia. Each deals with it in their own way.**

**Family members have differing reactions when the person is in a nursing home or hostel.**

**Sadness is the overwhelming emotion for relatives. When death comes to the resident, the grieving is nearly all done.**

**Relatives may act in a way of which you do not approve. Do not guess the reason; you can be wrong.**

**It is not a good idea to give advice to relatives on how to live their lives.**

**Your listening and understanding helps the relative cope with the day and gives you the satisfaction of knowing you have helped.**

**Relatives may benefit from counselling, joining a relatives support group or a relatives telephone network.**

# Effects on the family

Dementing illness affects every member of the family. Here are the stories of two families:

'The effects of Dad's illness are so gradual, we convince ourselves that his strange behaviour is due to business worries. After all, he is a loving husband and father and has always provided comfortably for my mother, brother and me.

Then one day the bank manager calls my mother. The house has to be sold to cover the repayments Dad hasn't made on a mortgage he took out without telling her.

For over a year he used the money to help 'the needy', and even though he opens the exclusive menswear shop he owns each morning, there is no stock to sell.

We move into a home unit; my mother works to pay the bills, Dad's debts, that come with every mail. Our friends are sympathetic but, I suppose not knowing what to say, keep away.

Mother is hurt when a longtime friend asks that Dad not visit because she finds it embarrassing.

Gradually my mother cuts herself off from life except for work and looking after Dad. I watch helplessly as my pretty, carefree, fifty-year-old Mum becomes weary and depressed and I cancel my wedding to stay with her.

Dad doesn't look any different and it is hard to realise that the Dad I knew no longer exists. I don't know how to relate to him—sometimes I find myself asking his advice as I always have; sometimes I treat him like a child. I cry a lot.

My young brother leaves university for the time being and is our strength. Even when the sadness and frustration get to us, he remains calm. He and I worry whether we might inherit Dad's disease but decide we don't want to know.

Dad goes to a nursing home a few weeks before he dies. Mother is the only one he recognises, and even though he has hardly spoken for months, he tells her 'Love you' each night when she visits.

I gaze at the pieces that were once my radio. I just can't take any more. He has to go to the nursing home! 'Fixing things' is his latest phase and the house is littered with appliances in various stages of disrepair.

Our marriage has been over for years; we live separate lives under the same roof. But when the tests confirm he is suffering from dementia I feel it is my responsibility to look after him.

Even though I have wonderful help from home care services, the nurse who comes to shower him, and two days a week at the day centre, I resent the time I have to spend looking after him. It is as though I am in a cage with no escape.

He often falls and helping him up exhausts me. Most nights he wakes after a nightmare or needs changing, and I haven't had a decent sleep for over a year. He is bad-tempered and always insists he is right even though what he says doesn't make sense.

My daughter blames me for putting him away. She can't believe her father's condition is permanent, even after several medical opinions. It upsets her to see him in this state and she seldom visits.

I visit him every few days in the nursing home, feeling angry that he has put me in a position of feeling guilty. I am sad to see him deteriorate to just a shell, yet relieved that I am free.

# Reactions of the family

The way that family members respond to the person with dementia often depends on the quality of the relationship they had with the person before he or she became demented. Each family member will react in their own way when their relative is admitted to a hostel or nursing home.

## *Participating in the caring*

When Eric's wife moves to the nursing home he continues to spend some time each day with her, sometimes taking her along when he calls on clients. He launders her clothes and is particular about her being well groomed.

Staff have mixed feelings: some feel he is dissatisfied with the way they care for her, some approve, and others are concerned that he is under stress.

Eric senses their attitudes but finds it difficult to explain that the relief of the main burden of caring has allowed him to spend more quality time with his wife.

He doesn't know how to tell them that every minute he can spend with this woman, his wife of thirty years, is precious. And while he understands their persistence in advising him to take a holiday— 'Leave her to us, we'll take care of her'—it adds to the strain.

### Unable to face the tragedy

As Mr Lee deteriorates, his sons cannot face the sadness of the weekly visit. As well, they want their children to remember their grandfather as he was. They do not come.

### Denying the illness

Mrs Paul's daughter is angry with her father for taking her mother to a dementia hostel. She moves her to a private nursing home. It is only when her mother wanders away and is lost for two days that she realises the seriousness of her mother's dementia.

### Sadness

The overwhelming emotion of families is sadness. The hardest part for relatives to bear is to see the disintegration of the person they once knew. They grieve. The mourning goes on day after day. When the person dies, although they are sad, it is almost an anticlimax. The grieving is done and sadness is tinged with relief for their relative's release and that they no longer need to watch the deterioration of a loved one.

# Giving advice

It is better not to give advice to relatives on how they should conduct their lives. What is right for you is often wrong for someone else.

Out of sympathy for relatives you might try to persuade them to take a holiday or advise them not to come to the unit for a day or two. Some may be relieved that you approve of them having a break. On the other hand, if you persist others, appreciating your concern, may stay away simply to please you. They then spend the time worrying about their relative, maybe phoning every few hours to check.

Make suggestions but do not persist with your advice.

### *Do not assume*

We often become so identified with the resident that we criticise families for acting in ways of which we do not approve. Seeking to understand, we often guess at the reason.

We can be wrong!

> Not knowing a woman has been in hospital for serious surgery, the supervisor phones to tell her that her husband is fretting and to chide her for not visiting more.
>
> ———
>
> A woman is accused by staff of selfishness for working, instead of looking after her dementing husband. The wife is trying to pay off her husband's debt in order to save their home.

### *Listen and understand*

Take notice of what family members tell you and try to understand their point of view.

Do not take complaints personally; relatives are not criticising you. Consider also the possibility that the complaint may be justified. Investigate and try to rectify the problem. Maybe something has particularly upset the relative. Encourage them to talk about it. Just having someone listen will help them through the day and you will feel satisfied that you have been of some assistance.

# Counselling

At times relatives benefit from discussing their concerns with a counsellor or in a support group. Provide them with the name and address of a social worker or counsellor who specialises in dementia, a carers' group or the Alzheimer's Association.

A support group within the nursing home or hostel is sometimes more helpful than an outside group.

## Family telephone network

In times of stress being in touch with someone in the same situation (even if only for an occasional chat) provides valuable support. Suggest the relatives in your unit form a telephone network—a list of phone numbers of those who agree to be contacted. Never give a relative's phone number or address without first asking permission.

# STAFF—CARING FOR YOURSELF

Caring for a number of people with dementia is a tiring and stressful occupation.

Doubts about our own mental health, our feelings and doubts about how we are coping with difficult situations often cause anxiety.

Release tension by:

—talking it over

—relaxing

—seeing the funny side

—leaving work worries behind

—exercising

—socialising

Be kind to each other. Credit yourself and each other with doing a worthwhile job.

## Care for yourself

The work of caring for a number of people in the advanced stages of dementia is a stressful occupation. Staff who work with elderly people are usually dedicated and caring and feel helpless and depressed to see loved residents slowly deteriorate.

We are sorry for, but often feel inadequate to comfort, grieving families. The strain of bad days in the unit, when anxiety is high and residents require more of our attention, adds to the pressure.

# We have doubts

### Am I getting dementia?

Working with dementing people makes us more aware of our own forgetfulness. We worry that it is the first sign of memory loss in ourselves.

Forgetting is normal: we all forget. We might have more important things on our minds, such as work pressures, a personal worry or the anticipation of an exciting event that distracts our thoughts.

My sixteen-year-old granddaughter phoned me, 'I am worried, I need to come to see you.'

> 'I think I am getting Alzheimer's,' she said, reeling off a string of things she was forgetting: forgetting to post letters, forgetting to meet her mother at an appointed time and place and so on. A formidable array of forgetting! But of course she was not becoming demented. She was in love. There was no room in her mind to remember day-to-day demands on her time. Her whole waking hours were filled with thoughts of the loved one.

It is not the forgetting that worries us. It is the remembering what it is we forgot. Memory loss is different. Memory loss is permanent and progressive and the person does not know what it is that is forgotten.

### Why bother?

Unfortunately, the benefits of what we achieve with the person with dementia are often not conspicuous. But stop to consider people in an environment where there is little or no stimulation or staff interaction. You see a silent, listless, vacant person often restrained in a chair or wandering aimlessly.

Do not expect too much. Rejoice in small gains. The violent woman regains her pleasant personality and speech when she is taken off physical and chemical restraint. The silent man remembers the words of songs when you encourage him to sing with the group. Your interest in learning about a woman's family may be rewarded by a smile and a cuddle. Even the hitherto withdrawn man who complains about his neighbour does so because he knows you understand. And any reaction is better than no reaction.

Families also are more content, reassured that you are interested in their loved relative.

### It seems dishonest

Are you a truthful person who believes it is wrong to agree with the seventy-year-old woman talking about her children at kindergarten? Or do you feel uncomfortable when you remind the woman who tells you she comes here for holidays each year that she is in a nursing home now? Should you tell the man who insists his wife is coming to see him that she died years ago?

This dilemma is a matter of conscience. Sometimes gentle truth is accepted by the dementing person but more often it is likely to confuse. The failing brain is telling one thing (the person's reality) and in being strictly truthful you may be emphasising another (your reality).

In order to work effectively with dementing people you need to be able to accept their reality. If this is difficult for you, talk to someone more experienced, or a counsellor who will help you sort it out.

## How do I answer relatives?

When relatives ask questions about the person's illness, we often feel that as staff we should know all the answers.

Do not be too embarrassed to say 'I don't know but I'll try to find out'. Or refer the person to a psychiatrist, social worker, psychologist or other health professional who specialises in dementia or in caring for the dementing person.

### What do I say when someone is dying?

It can be hard to respond to the grief of the relative of a person who dies or is dying. We wish we could do something to stop the hurt but we are often unable to find the right words. We may ignore them or try to cheer them up, neither of which is much comfort.

If you have this sort of difficulty, simply saying 'I'm sorry', or giving a hug or a squeeze of the hand, will convey your sympathy.

# It's really getting me down!

At times we all feel that working with dementing people gets us down. Some feel this more than others. You may feel inadequate. You might believe that you do not have enough knowledge. You might feel that you could do more with the dementing person if only you had the time.

Or has the system got you beaten? Nursing home schedules not appropriate for mobile dementing residents? Staff cuts, made to reduce the cost of running the unit, may have increased your workload to an intolerable level. Are you frustrated by a system of regimentation that prevents you from interacting with the residents? Share your feelings with your colleagues or your supervisor or, if your feelings of sadness, frustration or anger overwhelm you, seek counselling.

It is better not to confide your dissatisfactions to relatives as this not only adds to their burden but may also shake their confidence in you and the competence of the unit.

# Sometimes I feel angry

There may be times when you are so frustrated that you are tempted to 'take it out' on residents. Just as mothers may become exasperated with troublesome children and ignore or hit them, you may find yourself treating elderly residents in a similar way.

Almost without realising it you may take no notice when they call, forget to take them to meals or remove the meal uneaten. You may even 'forget' to toilet or change the person who is wet or soiled, or you may tie them into the bed or sedate them to prevent them from wandering out and annoying you. You might find an excuse to stop the resident from joining an excursion or staying overnight with his family.

If this is happening apply for some recreation leave; talk over your feelings with an experienced professional or consider asking for a transfer out of the unit.

# Why don't I like Mr Smith?

Do you feel kindly and affectionate towards most residents but dislike one person for a reason you cannot explain? Are you continually irritated by a particular relative?

You do not feel this way on purpose. Possibly the disliked person reminds you of someone with whom you had an unsatisfactory emotional relationship in the past. It may be an older relative that you now have strong feelings about. If you are stressed by caring for an elderly relative in your private life, it is usually better not to work with elderly people.

Talk to your supervisor or seek counselling to help you with these feelings.

# Releasing tension

Develop an awareness of the level of pressure you can tolerate without being adversely affected. If you are stressed and 'nervy', do something about it.

## *Talk it over*

Sharing your feelings helps to relieve the strain and often helps to clarify the reason for your tension.

The co-worker in whom you confide may be having the same difficulties. Tackle the problem together or, if she has solved the situation, you may benefit from her experience. Your supervisor or a person who has worked in the dementia field for some time has undoubtedly faced some of the difficulties you are experiencing. She may be able to help. Otherwise you may need to seek counselling.

## *Staff meetings and shorter shifts*

Some dementia units encourage staff to meet at regular intervals to discuss work problems and stresses.

In units where shorter shifts or longer breaks between shifts have been introduced, work stress and staff turnover has decreased.

### See the funny side

Keep your sense of humour. You experience lots of funny, even hilarious, moments working with people affected by dementia. Do not feel guilty if you find that you want to laugh. So long as you laugh with the person, they will enjoy the joke too. Save up your funny stories and share them with your colleagues.

### Relax

Attend a relaxation group until you have mastered the technique of relaxing your body. You will then be able to relax at will. Meditation is an excellent way to relax and get rid of all the tensions.

### Time out

Discipline yourself to take time out. Ask a co-worker to stand in for you when you feel overly tense. Find a quiet corner, relax or just sit and 'switch off' for a few minutes. You will handle your work more easily when you are composed.

Have meal and morning-tea breaks well away from the unit and the residents. If it is not possible for you to leave the premises, sit in the garden or find a quiet spot.

Take regular vacations. At least two holidays a year are necessary for the health and wellbeing of staff working with dementia.

### Don't take your work worries home

It is not always easy to leave work behind but for your peace of mind, be firm. Separate yourself emotionally and mentally from work as you walk out the door. Thinking and worrying achieves nothing for you or the resident, and eventually drains your enthusiasm for the job.

### Exercise and recreation

Exercise and recreation are both necessary for your health, wellbeing and balance in your working life. Find a hobby or sport that interests you and gives you pleasure. If you are married or sharing a house, do not spend all your spare time catching up on the housework. Plan definite times to enjoy yourself with family and friends.

### One stress at a time

If you have emotional problems in your home or private life, you are well advised to seek an occupation that is less stressful. Seek help to solve your problems and if you enjoy working with dementing people, return to it later.

### Cooperation

Cooperation—working as a team and sharing the load—relieves work tensions. Develop trust in each other and help out when a co-worker is having difficulties or feeling down.

### Socialise

Socialising binds a team together. Have a weekly cup of coffee at the local restaurant, an occasional picnic or theatre party. In a relaxed atmosphere you will get to know another side of the person you work with.

### Support each other

Be kind to yourself and to each other. What you are doing is worthwhile and you deserve credit for a job well done.

Recognise your value. A little mutual back-patting does not go astray and works wonders for the self-esteem.

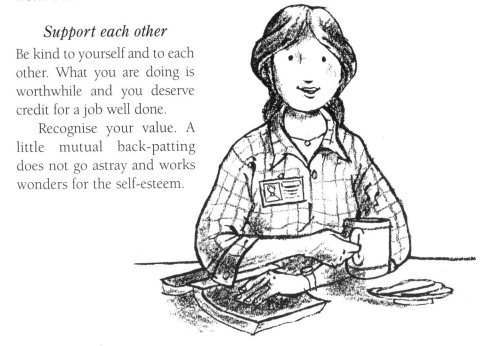

# Personal profile

NAME <u>Ruth White</u>　　　AGE <u>69</u>　　　DATE OF BIRTH <u>3/8/1921</u>

PREFERRED NAME <u>Ruth or 'Nan'</u>

SPOUSE'S NAME OR NICKNAME <u>Pete</u>

NAME, ADDRESS, RELATIONSHIP OF CARER <u>Jenny Green</u>

<u>4 Small St, Oldtown</u>　　　PHONE <u>823 4520</u>

daughter

CHILDREN, GRANDCHILDREN (living?)
Jenny m. John – Karen, Tracy, Peter

Paul m. June – Jennifer, Tony

BROTHERS, SISTERS (alive?)
Frieda lives in England

Ivy – sees her frequently – a very close relationship

WHERE BORN, EARLY HISTORY
Born Ashfield happy family. Attended Ashfield Primary School, then Sydney Girls High School.

Played competition tennis.

Father died 1970. Mother died 1968 – talks about parents

ADULT LIFE (marriage, children, significant happenings)
Occupation – hairdresser. Married Pete during WWII. Both served in R.A.A.F. in Victoria. Remembers Pete going to Canada to train as a pilot before they married.

Children both born in Victoria.

Paul nearly died from pneumonia when he was 5 years old

Was bridesmaid for Frieda and Ivy.

**HOBBIES, INTERESTS, SOCIAL CONTACTS** (including clubs, groups)

Used to knit and crochet – still likes to knit in a sort of way. Played tennis and bowls president of ................... Bowls club. She and Pete had many friends – liked to dance and play piano.

**PLACES LIVED**

Ashfield. Bowral as a teenager when parents bought a farm. Ballarat, Vic. Back to Sydney in 1950, lived in same house in Ryde all married life.

**PLACES VISITED**

Northern Territory – talks about Ayers Rock, Darwin, Fiji, Noumea, Washington, Los Angeles, U.S.A., England – recognises pictures of these places

**BEHAVIOUR PERSONALITY** (any recent changes?)

Happy, loving person loved by everyone. Lately has become suspicious and irritable, but mostly just delightfully vague. Often mixes up people. Sometimes thinks she's in Victoria. Phones daughter repeatedly mostly early hours of morning.

**OTHER SIGNIFICANT FACTORS—LIKES, DISLIKES**

Plays cards. Likes to chat. Can still play one or two pieces on piano.

Very particular about her appearance. Often thinks children are young.

| J. Jones S.W. | 20.4.1990 |
| --- | --- |
| SIGNED | DATE |

# Problem-solving approach

The following is the process of solving the problem with Mr Bass on page 99.

Mr Bass had become increasingly aggressive over several weeks shortly after his arrival at the nursing home. Sedation had had little effect. Two solutions were being considered: transfer to a psychiatric hospital for treatment or to a dementia unit with staff and facilities to deal with serious behaviour problems.

The problem-solving approach was applied to the problem:

| | |
|---|---|
| **THE PROBLEM** | Increasing aggression and sometimes hitting out at staff. |
| **WHOSE PROBLEM?** | Mr Bass who was increasingly upset and alienated from residents and staff. |
| | Staff who had become frightened of him. |
| **DESIRABLE OUTCOME** | Aggressive behaviour to cease. |
| **TOLERABLE OUTCOME** | Some decrease in undesirable behaviour. |
| | |
| **ASSESSMENT** | The person: A search of Mr Bass's personal profile indicated that he had no living relatives; he was the youngest of five children. The family had been devout Catholics with three sisters becoming nuns and one brother a member of the Marist Order. The independent hostel where he had previously lived reported that he was a quiet person who 'got on well' with staff and other residents, although he had spent a lot of time in his own company. He had been a regular attender at 6 am Mass at the church next door to the hostel. |
| **THE SITUATION** | Two nurses remembered that Mr Bass's aggression had first surfaced when he was refused breakfast after the weekly Mass in the nursing home. When they explained that he had eaten breakfast no more than an hour ago he did not believe them, but when given a piece of toast or a biscuit, he would take no more than a bite then throw it |

away. Staff could not identify a pattern for his other outbursts.

**STRATEGY**

**1** Because of Mr Bass's strong ties with his religion, it was decided to consult the priest who, after discussion with staff, suggested that one of the problems might be Mr Bass's lifelong habit of not eating from 12 midnight until after morning Mass, a practice that had once been a requirement of the Church.

*The problem has changed*—it is probably now a reaction to Mr Bass's *memory* of hunger (even the language has changed).

**2** On the following Sunday, half of Mr Bass's breakfast was set aside until after he came from Mass: he accepted it and ate with a smile. This practice was continued and there were no more outbursts on Sundays.

**3** Once they knew the reason for Mr Bass's aggression, staff attitude changed and as a result his aggressive behaviour gradually ceased altogether.

So what had happened here?

By using the problem-solving approach, the problem changed from one of aggression, with a fairly severe management plan to deal with Mr Bass's reaction, to a *memory* of extreme hunger and needing to eat as soon as possible after Mass. The second problem was the attitude of staff towards him. Because of his increasing irascibility, they tended to ignore him or react to him in a combative manner and he retaliated once or twice by trying to attack a nurse.

Once the real problem was identified the situation had a very simple solution, satisfactory to both Mr Bass and staff. But had staff acted on the first identified problem, Mr Bass would have been transferred for treatment to a psychiatric or other institution.

# The seven rules of caring for the home carer

Caring for a person with dementia is a physical and emotional ordeal for the home caregiver. If you are to survive reasonably well there are rules you must follow. Following these rules will make life easier. Not easy, but easier.

### RULE 1: KEEP WELL

Rest as much as you are able if you do not feel well. Do not put off going to the doctor because you don't have time. Eat sensibly. Get at least a few good nights' sleep every week. Exercise. Walk, garden, play a sport or join an exercise class. Don't give up your hobbies and leisure activities, plan to fit them in somehow.

### RULE 2: TAKE ADVANTAGE OF ALL THE HELP YOU CAN GET

Include your family in the caring. Have a family conference, encourage the family to find out as much information as they can about dementia. Ask them to share some of the caring. Exploit every type of respite service available; day caring either at a centre or in a home; book the person in to a nursing home or hostel so that you can have a planned break; join a support group and go to meetings. In other words, build up a network of support and supporters.

### RULE 3: CONFIDE IN OTHERS

We often try to hide the fact that someone close to us has dementia. We are embarrassed or a bit fearful of how others will react. Be upfront. Tell people what is wrong; in most cases they will understand and be sympathetic. For example, tell the local shopkeeper and your regular tradesmen. You can avoid all sorts of difficult situations if you do this. And it helps to educate others about dementia.

### RULE 4: DON'T DO MORE THAN YOU CAN MANAGE

Looking after someone with dementia is time consuming. You must learn to let some things go. Your visitors won't mind if the floor isn't polished or the furniture not dusted or your garden not weeded. They come to see you, not your kitchen floor. Get into the habit of occasionally not seeing the dust or the weeds.

### RULE 5: DON'T FEEL GUILTY

Don't dwell on whether you are doing enough for the person you are caring for, or think you should do better. Or that you aren't patient enough. We all have a tendency to think there must be something more we can do, or that if we had done something differently, things wouldn't be so bad. That is unlikely. We can't always be the sweet patient carer that we believe we should be.

### RULE 6: MAKE A PLAN

Try to plan your life ahead for six months. Yes, I know you don't even have enough time to think about tomorrow let alone six months forward. Well, it will just take 30 minutes of your time. Sit down when the house is quiet with a pen and paper and write down your plan. And stick to it. Your care plan might include one day each week just for yourself to go shopping or window shopping; visit friends; go to a film or stay at home and read a book, watch a video or just rest. It can give you a wonderful feeling to get a backlog of jobs done without interruption. Reward yourself when you keep to your plan, a hairdo, an afternoon at the club, a round of golf or your favourite chocolate. Go on, you can manage it!

Book a period of respite for the person you are caring for and take yourself off for a holiday or indulge yourself in some other way.

*It is so easy to feel totally defeated by the whole job of caring, and planning ahead will give you some control over what is happening in your life.*

### RULE 7: KNOW WHEN YOU HAVE HAD ENOUGH

There may come a time when you feel as though you just can't cope any more. Try not to force yourself to keep going. If you wear yourself out, who will be there to look after your loved one or protect their interests? What if you become ill or have a nervous breakdown? Don't wait for that to happen—don't become so exhausted and ill that you die before the disabled person does. There comes a time for many of us when we do need to consider residential care for the person with dementia.

Accept this graciously. If you feel badly about it, talk it over with a counsellor.

One carer's simple plan:

| | |
|---|---|
| **TUESDAYS** | Care Centre day. I'll do some chores that I haven't been able to find time for: I need to clean out the cupboard and put away the winter clothes. |
| **THURSDAYS** | Respite worker at home. Go to exercise class and have lunch at local café. |
| **ALTERNATE FRIDAYS** | Friend or daughter looks after him—go shopping or go to film. If they can stay for day, visit friends. |
| **LAST FRIDAY OF MONTH** | Attend carers' group (where … is cared for). |
| **NOVEMBER 7 TO 28** | Booked to go on week's holiday while … is in respite care. Second week, I'll just please myself what to do. |

This is actually a plan made by a female carer. Every time she achieved a part of her plan, she rewarded herself with a chocolate or buying herself a small gift or even indulging herself with a long leisurely phone call to a friend. She also got into the habit of praising herself for a job well done.

# Carer support organisations

## ALZHEIMER'S ASSOCIATION
Branches in capital cities throughout Australia. Support groups meet throughout Australia and New Zealand

**1800 639 331**
This toll-free number connects you to the association in your State or Territory.

## CARER'S ASSOCIATION
Support groups meet throughout Australia.

**Toll-free numbers**
ACT 1800 242 636
NSW 1800 817 023
NT 1800 242 636
Qld 1800 017 223
SA 1800 815 549
Tas. 1800 242 636
Vic. 1800 242 632
WA 1800 242 636

*Other support organisations*
## ADVOCACY SERVICES
These services are available in each state and territory and are listed in the phone book.

## COUNCIL ON THE AGEING (COTA)
Services are available in all states and are listed in the phone book.

**Toll-free numbers**
NSW 1800 449 102
SA 1800 182 324
Vic. 1800 136 381

## DEPARTMENT OF HEALTH AND FAMILY SERVICES
Contact the office in your capital city.

**Toll-free numbers in each state and territory.**

## CENTRELINK
The department has regional offices. Social work assistance is available through these offices.

Call **13 23 00** for the cost of a local call from anywhere in Australia.

### DEPARTMENT OF VETERANS' AFFAIRS

The department has offices in all states and territories which are listed in the phone book.

### AGED CARE ASSESSMENT TEAMS

These teams are available in geographic areas. Contact teams through your doctor, a community centre in your local district or the hospital social work department.

### GUARDIANSHIP TRIBUNAL

Guardianship Tribunals have been established in New South Wales, Victoria and South Australia. The ACT has an Office of the Community Advocate. In other states similar legal authorities act to appoint guardians.

### HOME CARE SERVICE

Contact Aged Care Assessment Teams (ACAT), district home care agencies, community and neighbourhood centres, and hospital social work departments.

### HOME NURSING SERVICE

For referral for assistance with home nursing, contact the Nursing Service direct, a medical practitioner, ACAT or community centre.

### INDEPENDENT LIVING CENTRES

These centres are situated in each state and are listed in the phone book.

### MEALS ON WHEELS

Contact local councils, community centres, neighbourhood centres, district hospitals ACATs and social work departments.

### MEMORY DISORDERS CLINICS

These are attached to some large public hospitals with referrals mainly through general medical practitioners and outpatients departments.

### SOCIAL WORK DEPARTMENTS

All public hospitals and some private hospitals have a social work service.

# List of terms

**affect**  the personality, emotions and mood

**agnosia**  inability to comprehend the meaning of what is seen, heard, touched, smelled or tasted

**agraphia**  writing difficulties

**alexia**  reading difficulties

**anomia**  loss of capacity to name objects or find the correct words to express an idea

**aphasia**  difficulty in verbal expression and/or comprehension; inability to carry on a conversation

**apraxia**  inability to translate a thought into an appropriate action; despite knowing what it is she or he wants to do, the person is unable to organise and carry out the gesture or movement

**benign senescent forgetfulness**  ability to remember the essentials of day-to-day living, such as who and where the person is and even how to prepare a meal or feed the cat, but memory of recent events that do not matter, such as the name of the present prime minister or the day and date, may be patchy or imperfect (sometimes called 'benign dementia')

**body image**  knowledge of how the body looks, the position of the parts and how they relate to each other (including familiar objects such as a wedding ring or wallet)

**circumlocution**  'talking around' a subject; using several words or sentences to explain a word or simple idea

**cognition**  the intellectual capacity or faculty that directs thinking and association of ideas

**confabulation**  an explanation, fabricated by the dementing person to make sense of his or her confused world, that is fully believed by the teller and believable to the listener

**deficits**  physical and intellectual skills the person has difficulty with or can no longer perform; inappropriate behaviour and emotions

**delirium**  a mental disturbance usually of short duration, often associated with an infectious illness and characterised by confusion

**delusion**   a false idea, believed by the teller despite attempts at rational argument; sometimes with a bizarre quality and often obviously untrue

**dementia**   an organic degeneration of the brain manifested by loss of memory and other intellectual functions, and personality changes

**disorientation**   a state of mind in which the sense of time, direction and recognition are muddled

**dysgraphia**   see 'agraphia'

**dyslexia**   see 'alexia'

**dysphasia**   see 'aphasia'

**dyspraxia**   see 'apraxia'

**emotion**   expression of a feeling; emotions may be negative or positive, for example anger or pleasure

**hallucination**   a false perception in which the person sees, hears, smells, tastes and/or touches something that does not exist

**illusion**   a mistaken impression or idea due to misinterpretation of a real experience

**inertia**   inability to move or act spontaneously; often mistaken for lack of motivation in the dementing person

**initiative**   taking the first step oneself towards commencing an activity or starting a movement

**organic orderliness**   meticulous tidiness or re-ordering of possessions without apparent reason and often in a strange or unusual arrangement

**paranoia**   delusions of being persecuted or victimised; the person may irrationally accuse others of stealing or otherwise intending harm

**paraphasia**   the use of incorrect or senseless words, or the use of words in wrong combinations

**perception**   a conscious recognition of what is being heard, seen, touched or otherwise sensed

**perseveration**   persistent repetition of an activity, word or phrase, often without reason

**psychiatric symptoms**   symptoms of specific mental illnesses rather than symptoms of brain degeneration or intellectual disability; a person with dementia may also exhibit psychiatric symptoms, such as some forms of depression, delusions and hallucinations

**reality orientation** a process of reinforcing aspects of reality in an attempt to reduce the confusion of the world as the dementing person perceives it; it is most effectively employed by repeatedly naming persons, objects and places

**recall** remembering; reviving a memory

**reinforcement** employing pleasant experiences, praise, repetition and stimulation of the senses, to preserve the person's memory and life skills for as long as possible

**reminiscence** talking about or otherwise relating one's memories

**spatial ability** the ability to know where one's body is in space and in relation to people and objects in the environment; also the capacity to see how objects relate to each other—behind, under, above, and so on (also referred to as 'spatial sense' and 'spatial orientation')

**strengths** skills, intellectual capacities, appropriate behaviour and emotions retained by the person

**therapy** treatment aimed at improving or healing a physical or mental disorder; standard therapeutic procedures have little or no effect on dementia

**weaknesses** see 'deficits'

# Bibliography

*Aged Care Act 1997*, Principles, Commonwealth of Australia, 1997.

Alzheimer's Association NSW, *Newsletters*, July 1982–January 1999.

Alzheimer's Association National Conference proceedings, 1989–1997.

Berg, A., Welander, H.U. & Hallberg Ingalill, R., 'Nurses creativity, tedium and burnout during one year of clinical supervision and implementation of individually planned nursing care: Comparisons between a ward for severely demented patients and a similar control ward', *Journal of Advanced Nursing*, 20, 1994.

Bird, Michael, 'Pyscho-social rehabilitation for problems rising from cognitive deficits in dementia', in R. Hill, L. Backman & A. Stigsdotter Neeley (eds), *Cognitive Rehabilitation in Old Age*, Oxford University Press, London, 1998.

Bird, Michael, Llewellyn-Jones, R., Smithers, H., et al., 'Challenging behaviours in dementia: A project of Hornsby/Ku-ring-gai Hospital', *Australian Journal on Ageing*, 17 (1), 1998.

Brodaty, H., 'Minimal brain damage in the adult. II Early dementia', *Patient Management*, August 1988, p. 127.

Brodaty, H., 'Guide to medical jargon', *The Dementia Educator*, Alzheimer's Association NSW, 1997.

Brodaty, H. & Griffin, D., 'The management of dementia', *Modern Medicine of Australia*, September 1981, p. 25.

Burnside, I., 'Content about Alzheimer's disease in nursing curricula: A dire need', *Proceedings IV International Meeting, Alzheimer's Disease International*, 1988.

Butler, R., 'The challenge of dementia' (opening address), *Proceedings IV International Meeting, Alzheimer's Disease International*, 1988.

Commonwealth/State/Territory Program, *Home and Community Care Program, National Guidelines*, Australian Government Publishing Service, Canberra, 1992.

Commonwealth/State Working Party on Nursing Home Standards, June 1987, *Living in a Nursing Home; Outcome Standards for Australian Nursing Homes*, Australian Government Publishing Service, Canberra, 1987.

Doyle, C., *Evaluation of Innovative Dementia Programmes: A Short Review*, National Centre for Health Program Evaluation, Monash University and Melbourne University, Melbourne.

Doyle, S., 'Pyschotropic drug use among older people', *Lincoln Papers in Gerontology*, July 1993.

Drickhamer, M.A. & Lachs, M.S., 'Should patients with Alzheimer's disease be told of their diagnosis?', *The New England Journal of Medicine*, 1992, 326

Fleming, R. & Bowles, J., 'Special housing units for the confused and disturbed elderly', ADARDS Newsletter, 13, January/March 1987.

Freytag, K., Harrison, J., et al., *If Only I'd Known*, Transrubicon Pty Ltd ACA, 1986.

Geeves, M., 'New directions in staff education', *Proceedings IV International Meeting, Alzheimer's Disease International*, 1988.

Goldwasser, A., Auerbach, S. & Hawkins, S., 'Cognitive, affective and behavioural effects of reminiscence group therapy on demented elderly', *International Journal of Aging and Human Development*, 25, 1987.

Griffin, D., *Straight from the Heart, A Consumer's Eye View of Nursing Homes*, ADARDS, NSW.

Gwyther, L.P., *Care of Alzheimer's Patients: A Manual for Nursing Home Staff*, American Health Care Association, ADARDA, 1985.

Hall, G., Kirschling, M.V. & Todd, S., 'Sheltered freedom in an Alzheimer's unit in an ICF', *Geriatric Nursing* (USA), May/June 1986.

Hamilton-Smith, E., Hooker, D. & James, M., 'Granny is a bit strange: The medicalisation of dementia', paper to Annual Conference of Australian Sociological Association, 10–13, 1992.

Hoffman, S.B. & Kaplan, M. (eds), *Special Care Programs for People with Dementia*, Health Professions Press, Baltimore, 1996.

Holden, U.P. & Woods, R.T., *Reality Orientation*, Churchill Livingstone, London, 1982.

Jorm, A.F. & Henderson, A.S., *The Problem of Dementia in Australia* (3rd edn), Department of Health Housing and Community Services, Aged and Community Division, Canberra.

Kerr, P.E., *Identification of Nurses' Stress Engendered by Caring for Dementia Residents in Nursing Homes*, treatise completed as partial requirement of the Master of Community Health program, Faculty of Health Sciences, University of Sydney, 1993.

Kovach, C.R., 'Promise and problems in reminiscence research', *Journal of Gerontological Nursing*, 16 (4).

Kratiuk, S., Young, J., Rawson, G. & Williams, S., *A Double Jeopardy, a Report on Dementia in Clients of Non-English Speaking Backgrounds*, South Western Sydney Area Health Service, 1992.

Mace, N.L. & Rabins, P.V., *The 36-Hour Day*, John Hopkins University Press, 1983.

Mackenzie-Thurley, S., 'Nursing issues: Intimidation of the elderly in institutions', *Proceedings of the 21st Annual Conference*, Australian Association of Gerontology, 1986.

Ministerial Task Force on Pyschotropic Medication Use in Nursing Homes (1997), discussion paper, NSW Health, 1997.

Mitchell, K.R., Kerridge, I.H. & Lovat, T.J., *Bioethics and Clinical Ethics for Health Care Professionals*, Social Science Press, 1996.

National Institute of Aging, National Institutes of Health, Bethesda, Maryland, *Alzheimer's Disease* (pamphlet).

Reeve, W.A., 'The carer: Angry feelings in relation to the dementing person', *Geriaction* 6 (7), 1984.

'Restraint: Exploring the pathway between risks and rights', report on Canberra Conference, *Dementia Today*, March 1997.

Ronalds, C., et al., *'I'm Still an Individual': An Issues Paper*, Department of Community Services and Health, 1988.

Rosewarne, R., Opie, B.A., et al., 'Care needs of people with dementia and challenging behaviours living in residential facilities' (Summary Report 1996), in *Aged and Community Care Service Development and Evaluation Reports*, 29, Australian Government Printing Service, Canberra, 1997.

Sammut, A., *Working with Families of Dementia Sufferers*, Assessment and Management Seminar, Cumberland College of Health Sciences, September 1988.

Satir, V., *Self Esteem*, Celestial Arts, Berkeley, California, 1975.

Sherman, B., 'Self image and the psychiatrically disabled', *Proceedings of Seminar, International Year of the Disabled*, Burwood Municipal Council, 1981.

Sherman, B., An Ethnic Dementia Program; *Relatives, Lifestyles and Ethnic Issues* (pamphlet) 1988.

Sherman, B., 'Solving the problem: A planned response to strange and difficult behaviour and disruptive actions', *Proceedings of the Alzheimer's Association (Australia) 4th National Conference*, 1994.

Sherman, B., 'Therapy: Who benefits?, A critical evaluation of the routine use of psychological type "therapy" in dementia programmes', *Proceedings of the International Conference of Alzheimer's International*, Edinburgh, 1994.

Sherman, B., *Sex, Intimacy and Aged Care*, ACER Press, 1998.

Sherman, B. & Hunt, J., 'The development of a dementia hostel in a large institution', *Proceedings IV International Meeting Alzheimer's Disease International*, 1988.

Slater, E. & Roth, M., *Clinical Psychiatry*, 3rd edn, Baillieu, Tindell and Cassell, London, 1969.

Snowdon, J., Miller, R. & Vaughan, R., 'Behavioural problems in Sydney nursing homes', *International Journal of Geriatric Psychiatry*, ll, 1998.

Symington, Norma, *Living and Communicating with Confused People* (pamphlet), ed. Barbara Squires, 1986.

Trowbridge, R., 'The conceptual confusion of therapeutic recreation', *Therapy and Recreation Seminar Proceedings*, Monash University, Melbourne, 1988.

Unwin, David, 'More flexible programs to meet the needs of residents suffering from dementia', *VCA Hostels Futures Conference proceedings*, October 1988.

Welander, H.U., Hallberg, I.R. & Axelsson, N., 'Nurses' satisfaction with care and work at three care units for severely demented people', *Journal of Psychiatric and Mental Health Nursing*, 2, 1995.

Zgola, J.M., *Doing Things*, John Hopkins University Press, Baltimore, 1987.
Zoblicki, M., 'Successful ageing in a public nursing home', proceedings of the 25th Annual Conference of the Australian Association of Gerontology, Canberra.

**VIDEO**
'Dementia with Dignity', Eastway Communications, Sydney, 1994.

# Index

**A**

activities, 54, 82, 171,
    229–42
  concerts, 239
  craft, 238
  domestic chores, 231–2
  entertainment, 238
  familiar, 82
  free choice of, 230
  individual interests, 233
  intellectual, 237–9
  music, 238–9
  outings, 6, 240–1
  physical, 236–7
  program of, 234–41
  radio, listening to, 232
  reading, 231
  reluctance to participate
    in, 114–17, 241–2
  reminiscing, 20, 233–4,
    237–8
  singing, 239
  structured, 230, 234–41
  television, watching, 232
aggression, 7, 15, 63–4,
    101–8
  anecdotes of, 25, 66–7,
    106–8
  anger and, 101–2
  management of, 103–6,
    256–7
  medication for, 106
  prevention of, 105
  reasons for, 103–4
  between residents, 67
agitation, 51, 121–3
  and change, 175
  evening, 122–3
  mealtime, 131
  *see also* anxiety
agnosia, 263
agraphia, 263

AIDS, 12
aids, 184–5
alcoholism, 12
alexia, 263
Alzheimer's Associations,
    179, 183, 186, 191,
    196, 247
Alzheimer's disease, 5–6,
    11–12, 51, 84
anger *see* aggression
anomia, 263
  anxiety associated with
  anticipation, 26
  change, 25
  confusion, 23, 25, 28
  coordination difficulties,
    37
  delusions, 45, 163–4
  fear of others, 45
  hallucinations, 45,
    164–5
  memory loss, 22
  not understanding, 34
  restriction and restraint,
    51
  sexual frustration, 133–9
  speech and word
    difficulty, 34
  strange surroundings, 53
  task failure, 39
  word difficulties, 34
aphasia, 263
appearance, 6, 84, 227
apraxia, 263
attention seeking, 108–11
  reasons for, 109
  renaming, 109
attitudes,
  cultural, 65, 128, 196
  family, 196, 211, 222–4,
    243–5
  staff, 86–7, 219, 248–53

**B**

barriers to communication,
    145–6
behaviour,
  changes in, 57
  institutional, 220
  problem, 15, 27–8, 57,
    63–4, 88–143
  symptomatic, 89–90
  *see also* personality
    changes
benign senescent
  forgetfulness, 263
blaming family, 210
body image, 263
body language, 148, 153
boredom, 124
brain failure, 11
  *see also* Alzheimer's
    disease; dementia

**C**

Carer Pension, 192
Carers' Association, 179,
    186, 190–1
caring, 179–253
  for families, 242–7
  at home, 179–94
  in hostel or nursing
    home, 195–253
  for primary carer,
    179–80
  for staff, 247–53
catastrophic reaction, 20,
    65–6, 116, 136–7,
    143, 177, 200, 202,
    220, 241
chairs, 184–5, 214
change, 174–8
  anxiety with, 53
  handling, 174–8

reactions to, 175
choice, 86, 176–7, 230
circumlocution, 263
clocks, 27
clothing, 84, 120–1, 182
cognition, 55, 263
communicating, 17, 29–34,
    144–57
  acquired language, 33–4
  asking questions, 20–1,
    150
  by body language, 148,
    153
  by facial expressions,
    148, 153
  hearing, 151–2
  listening, 151
  misunderstanding, 6, 17,
    29–31
  picking up clues, 152–3
  showing, 149
  speaking, 30–4, 147–8
  using statements, 151
communication difficulties,
    29–34, 145–6
comprehension, 31
concentration, 235–6
confabulation, 17, 43, 46–9,
    165, 263
  as explanation, 46–7
  to maintain identity,
    79–80
confusion, 17, 23–9
  about objects, 27–8,
    36–7
  about people, 24
  about place, 24–5
  about time, 25–7
  anxiety about, 23, 28
  and change, 25, 175–6
  and living alone, 29
coordination difficulties, 17,
    34–42
  and dressing, 35
  and getting started, 38–9
  and learning, 40
  and perception, 36, 41
  and sitting, 40–1

and standing, 41
and tasks, 37–8
and thoughts and
    actions, 34–42
and walking, 41–2
Creutzfeldt-Jakob's disease,
    12
cues, 17, 21–2, 38–9
cultural influences, 49

D
day care see respite care
death, 141–3, 249–50
deficits, 263
delirium, 263
delusions, 17, 43–4, 163–4,
    264
  of persecution, 44
  as reaction to change,
    211
  responding to, 45
  treatment of, 46
dementia, 10–15, 264
  Alzheimer's disease, 5–6,
    11–13
  brain failure, 8
  characteristics of, 14–15,
    17
  deterioration, 13, 64
  incurable, 13
  multi-infarct, 13
  myths about, 5–9
  progression of, 13
  stages of, 13–14
dementia unit,
  atmosphere of, 212
  environment, 212–18
  furnishings of, 212–16
  lifestyle in, 218–242
  and links with world,
    216–17
  location markers in, 172,
    215–16
  mirrors in, 84–5, 215
  moving to, 124–5,
    195–203
  personal possessions in,
    82–3, 117–21,

212–16
personal space in, 213
pets in, 228
relatives and, 204–5,
    222–4, 222–5, 228–9
routine in, 219
settling in, 172, 177,
    203–11
staff of, 202, 221
teamwork in, 221–2
telephones in, 218
visitors to, 227
dementing person see
    person with dementia
depression, 60–2
  assessment of, 60, 211
  and dementing illness,
    12, 60
  and mental illness, 60–2,
    264
  as reaction, 39, 61–2,
    211
  treatment of, 61–2
diagnosis, 180–1
discussion groups, 237–8
disorientation, 264
Domiciliary Nursing Care
    Benefit, 192
drugs see medication
dysgraphia, 264
dyslexia see alexia
dysphasia see aphasia
dyspraxia see apraxia

E
eating, 127–33
  agitation and, 131
  aids for, 129, 185
  appetite, 129
  atmosphere, 127
  choice of food, 128
  disruptive behaviour,
    132
  eating alone, 133
  feeding, 130
  food habits and tastes,
    128–9
  hunger, 130–1

messing, 132
spilling, 131
emotion, 155, 264
emotional reactions, 62–7,
    208–11
    anecdotes of, 66–7
    catastrophic, 20, 65–6,
        116, 136–7, 143,
        177, 200, 202, 220,
        241
    cultural factors in, 65
    extreme, 63, 210–11
    inappropriate, 63
    on moving, 197–8,
        208–11
    normal, 64
    reasons for, 64–5
    shallow, 63
eyesight, impaired, 235

**F**
families, 242–7
    and admission, 197
    blaming, 210
    counselling for, 246–7
    family groups, 247
    giving advice to, 245–6
    and illness, 243–4
    involvement with, 21, 69
    listening to, 246
    mixed feelings of, 210
    outings with, 241
    sadness of, 245
    seeking permission from,
        228–9
    support for, 247
financial matters, 191–3
    bank accounts, 192–3
    fees, 199
    power of attorney, 191,
        193
    see also pensions
forgetting, 18–22
friendships, 225–6
frustration see anxiety
functional assessment, 69,
    202
furniture, 125, 184–5
    see also dementia unit

**G**
grief, 139–43
    of families, 243–5
    of person with dementia,
        139–41
    as response to death,
        141–3
guardianship, 194
Guardianship Tribunal, 194,
    200, 262

**H**
habits, 73–4, 77
hallucinations, 17, 43–6,
    49, 164–5, 264
    anxiety about, 45
    and change, 211
    responding to, 45
    treatment of, 46
hearing, 30, 145, 235
hiding things, 117–18
hoarding, 119
holidays, 240
home carer, 126, 179–80,
    258–60
    counselling for, 190–1,
        196
    family assistance for,
        186, 188–9
    reactions of, 159, 196,
        211
    rest for, 126, 180, 187–9
    support for, 180, 185–6
    support groups for, 179,
        191, 261–2
home help, 186
home nursing, 186
hospitalisation, 178, 201
hostel see dementia unit
humour, 78–9
    among staff, 252
Huntington's disease, 12

**I**
identity, 68–87
    distortion of, 72–3
    loss of, 71
    survival of, 72–4

ways to confirm, 74–5,
    78–87
illusion, 264
incontinence, 125, 181–2
independence, 39, 87, 129
inertia, 264
initiative, 38, 264
institutional behaviour, 220
institutionalisation, 220
interpreters, 33–4

**L**
language, 30–4, 156–7
    body, 148, 153
    loss of, 30–4
laughter, 63, 226
learning, 40
legal matters, 191, 193–4
    competence, 193
    enduring power of
        attorney, 193–4
    guardianship, 194
Lewy body disease, 11–12
life roles, 73–6, 82
listlessness, 57–60
    combating, 59–60
    reasons for, 58
    and stimulation, 59–60
    as symptom of
        depression, 60
'looking for love and care',
    108–11
losing things, 117–18

**M**
masturbation, 137–8
medication,
    for delusions and
        hallucinations, 46
    for depression, 61–2
    and difficult behaviour,
        92
    for sleeplessness, 123
    therapeutic, 116
    on transfer to nursing
        home, 201
memory, prompting, 17,
    20–2

memory loss, 9, 17–22
  anxiety about, 20, 22
  degrees of, 18–19
modelling, 167–9
money, 83, 200
mood changes, 9, 15, 60–2
move to nursing home or
  hostel, 195–203
  choosing unit, 198–9
  cultural attitudes to, 196
  documents, 202–3
  family attitudes to, 197
  involving the person,
    197
  making decision, 195–8
  medication during, 201
  preparation for, 199–200
  refusal to go, 200–1
  transferring from
    hospital, 201–2
multi-infarct dementia, 13
music, 21
myths about people with
  dementia, 5–9

N
native language, 33–4,
  156–7
negative reactions, 114,
  116–17
noise, 239–40
non-cooperation, 63,
  114–17
nursing home see dementia
  unit

O
organic orderliness, 264
organisations, support,
  261–2
outings, 6, 240–1
overprotection, 228
P
paranoia, 264
paraphasia, 264
Parkinson's disease, 12, 109,
  131

pensions,
  Carer Pension, 192
  collection of, 192–3
  Domiciliary Nursing
    Care Benefit, 192
  special benefit, 192
  and transfer to unit, 203
perception, 36, 41, 264
perseveration, 264
person with dementia,
  16–54
  common characteristics
    of, 17
  identity of, 68–87
  relating to, 28, 69
  retained life roles of,
    73–6
  sense of humour of,
    78–9
  as unique individual,
    2–3, 68–87
personal possessions, 82–3,
  117–21
  clothing, 120, 226–7
  as confirmation of
    identity, 7, 82–3
  in dementia unit, 7,
    117–21
  packing, 200
  toilet articles, 226
personal profile, 70–1, 203,
  254–5
personality changes, 15,
  55–7
pets, 228
Pick's disease, 11–12
pilfering, 117–19
power of attorney, 181, 191
praise, 20, 37, 39, 42, 87,
  170–1
privacy, 21, 87
problem behaviour, 88–143
  at mealtime, 130–2
  medication for, 92
  prevention of, 93
  refusing medication, 116
  reluctance to participate,
    114–17, 241–2

response to, 93–7,
    112–14
  strategy for, 97–100
  what is it?, 91–2
psychiatric symptoms, 264

Q
questions, asking, 20–1,
  150

R
reading, 31, 231
reality orientation, 265
recall, 265
reflecting, 154–5
regimentation, 220
reinforcement, 169–74
  definition of, 169, 265
  praise as, 170–1
  repetition as, 171–2
  use of senses for, 173–4
relationships, 56–7
  personal, 158–9
  working, 157–62
religious services, 240–1
reminiscence, 265
reminiscing, 20, 22
repetitiveness, 77, 111–14
residential facility see
  dementia unit
respite care, 189–90
  day care, 189
  nursing home or hostel,
    189–90
restraint, 228–9
  see also medication
risk taking, 228–9
rummaging, 117–19
  management of, 120–1

S
second childhood, 1
sedation, 124, 210
self see identity; person with
  dementia
self-esteem, 22, 39, 72
  diminished, 72

senses, 21–2, 173–4
settling into unit, 203–11
  adapting, 206–8
  family reactions, 211
  first day, 206
  new resident's reactions,
    208–211
  unpacking, 205
  welcome, 204–5
sexual behaviour, 133–9
sexual harassment, 139
shrewdness, 9
sight *see* eyesight
sitting, difficulties with,
    40–1
skills,
  learning, 40
  loss of, 34–5
  maintaining, 235
  and non-coordination,
    35
  retained, 19–20
sleep, 123–6
  encouraging, 123–4
  interrupted, 125
  medication for, 123
  pattern reversal, 125–6
sleeplessness, 121–6
spatial ability, 265
staff, 247–53
  attitudes of, 86, 161
  caring for self, 247–8
  concerns of, 248–51
  in dementia unit, 202,
    221
  and relatives, 159–60,
    211, 222–4, 245–6,
    249–50
  releasing tension of,
    251–3
  support for, 251–3
  as team, 221–2
  training, 221
standing difficulties, 41
strengths, 265
suspiciousness, 9, 44,
    117–8
symbolism, 153–4

**T**
taking risks, 228–9
television,
  and chairbound resident,
    232
therapy, 265
time, 25–7

**V**
vascular dementia, 11
vision, tunnel, 235
  *see also* eyesight,
    impaired
visitors, 24, 227
volunteers, 110–11

**W**
walking, 41–2, 49–52
  aids for, 184–5
  alone, 51
  areas for, 7
  difficulties, 41, 184–5
    aids for, 42, 184–5
    assistance with,
      41–2
  excessive, 17, 51, 53
  as exercise, 182–3
  limiting, 50–1, 54
  pacing, 51
  patterns of, 50
  as reaction, 51
  reasons for, 51
  restraint and, 50–1
  stress driven, 51
wandering, 17, 49–50,
    52–4, 183
  aimless, 52
  away, 52
  and becoming lost, 7, 52
  identification for those,
    53, 183
  security for those, 53
weaknesses *see* deficits
words, 17, 29–34, 152, 172
  *see also* communicating
worker skills, 144–78
  communicating, 144–57
  handling change, 174–8

making relationships,
    157–62
modelling, 167–9
reinforcement, 169–74
world, 162–7
  of confabulations, 165
  delusional, 163–4
  distorted, 166–7
  hallucinatory, 164–5
  of the past, 163
  'real world,' 162–3,
    165–6
writing, 32